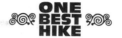

**ONE BEST HIKE**

# GRAND CANYON

D0972305

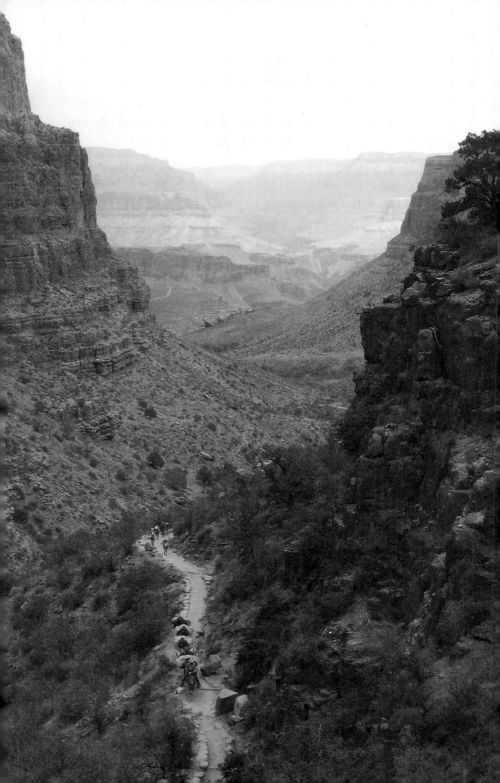

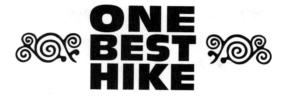

# GRAND CANYON

**Everything you need to know
to successfully hike from
the rim to the river
—and back**

## Elizabeth Wenk

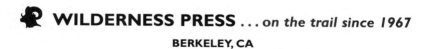

**WILDERNESS PRESS** ... *on the trail since 1967*

BERKELEY, CA

**One Best Hike: Grand Canyon**

**1st EDITION 2010**

Copyright © 2010 by Elizabeth Wenk

Cover photos copyright © 2010 by the author
Interior photos, except where noted, by the author
Maps and figures: Elizabeth Wenk and Larry B. Van Dyke
Cover design: Larry B. Van Dyke
Interior design: Andreas Schueller and Larry B. Van Dyke
Editor: Laura Shauger

ISBN 978-0-89997-491-0

Manufactured in the United States of America

Published by:  **Wilderness Press**
**1345 8th Street**
**Berkeley, CA 94710**
**(800) 443-7227; FAX (510) 558-1696**
**info@wildernesspress.com**
**www.wildernesspress.com**

Visit our website for a complete listing of our books and for ordering information.

Distibuted by Publishers Group West

*Front cover photos: Top:* Descending below Ooh Aah Point on the South Kaibab Trail; *Middle:* Walls of Coconino Sandstone rising above the Bright Angel Trail (near 1.5-Mile Resthouse); *Bottom:* Descending below Cedar Ridge on the South Kaibab Trail
*Back cover photos: Top:* View from Mather Point; *Bottom:* Ribbon Falls
*Frontispiece:* A mule train approaches Jacobs Ladder on the Bright Angel Trail.

To Eleanor and Sophia,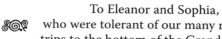
who were tolerant of our many research
trips to the bottom of the Grand Canyon

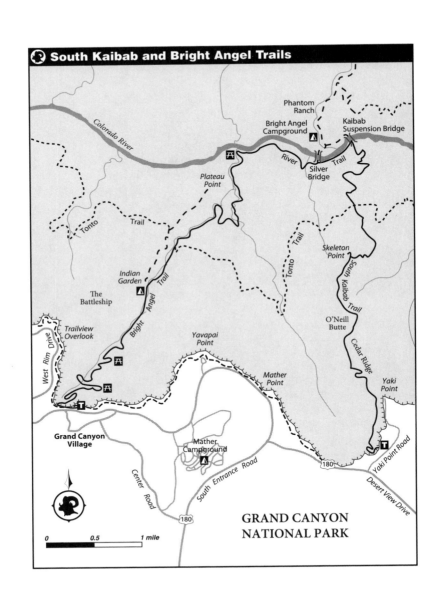

# South Kaibab and Bright Angel Trails

Colorado River

Phantom Ranch

Bright Angel Campground

Kaibab Suspension Bridge

River Trail

Silver Bridge

Plateau Point

Tonto Trail

Skeleton Point

Tonto Trail

Indian Garden

South Kaibab Trail

The Battleship

O'Neill Butte

Trailview Overlook

West Rim Drive

Bright Angel Trail

Cedar Ridge

Yavapai Point

Yaki Point

Mather Point

Grand Canyon Village

Mather Campground

South Entrance Road

180

Center Road

180

Yaki Point Road

Desert View Drive

**GRAND CANYON NATIONAL PARK**

0        0.5        1 mile

# CONTENTS

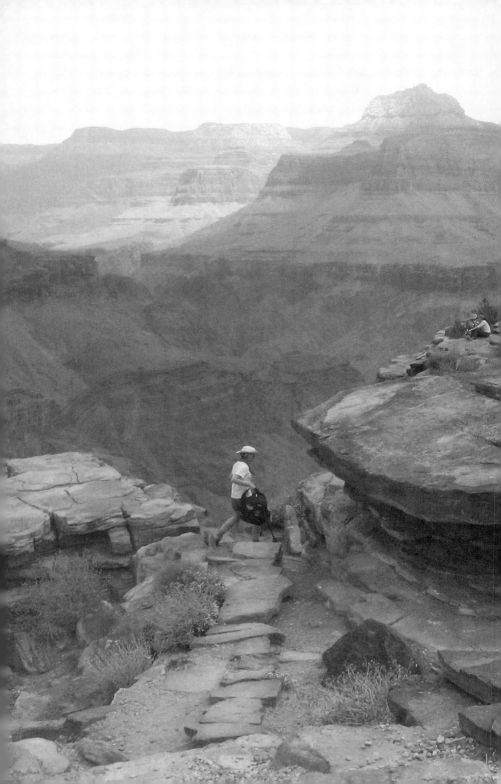

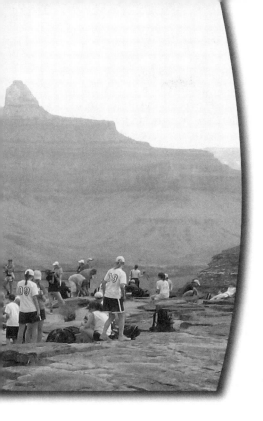

# 1
# Introduction

*"Stand at some point on the brink of the Grand Canyon where you can overlook the river, and the details of the structure, the vast labyrinth of gorges of which it is composed, are scarcely noticed; the elements are lost in the grand effect, and a broad, deep, flaring gorge of many colors is seen. But stand down among these gorges and the landscape seems to be composed of huge vertical elements of wonderful form."*
—John Wesley Powell,
*Explorations of the Colorado River and Its Canyons*

The Grand Canyon is one of the most recognizable natural features in the world: It earns a spot as one of the seven natural wonders of the world and is the best-known national park in North America. Five million people visit the Grand Canyon each year to enjoy the incomprehensibly grand views from the rim. However, as John Wesley Powell candidly wrote in 1875, you haven't really visited the Grand Canyon until you descend below the rim.

Each time I visit the Grand Canyon and stop at my first rim vista point, I anticipate the indescribably grand view, sit down, and stare in disbelief at the landscape. Can this place really exist? But the view satisfies me for only a short period of time; the rim views have an aerial feel and I want to be on the ground exploring. As I stare at the canyon, my mind begins to travel downward, tracing side canyons, following plateaus, and peering toward the river.

*Opposite and above:* Enjoying the view from Plateau Point

1

Before long my legs begin to twitch—at least figuratively—wishing to explore the intricacies of the landscape. In a mountainous wilderness, many people are motivated to hike to a summit to enjoy an otherwise unattainable vista. There are equally hidden vistas buried deep in the canyon: the walls of the Inner Gorge, the views of the inner canyon buttes once you are among them, mesas that merge with the landscape until you are below the rim, and of course the raging river. The landscape feels much more complex once you are in it, rather than looking down on it.

Therefore, don't allow yourself the complacency of sitting on the rim, enjoying the splendid panoramas and believing that you have "seen" the Grand Canyon. If you have ever stared at a view of the Grand Canyon—even if only a picture of the view—consider challenging yourself to descend to the bottom of the canyon. The two well-maintained trails, termed corridor trails, descending from the South Rim of the Grand Canyon, the Bright Angel Trail and the South Kaibab Trail allow tens of thousands of hikers to "see" the inner canyon and reach the Colorado River each year.

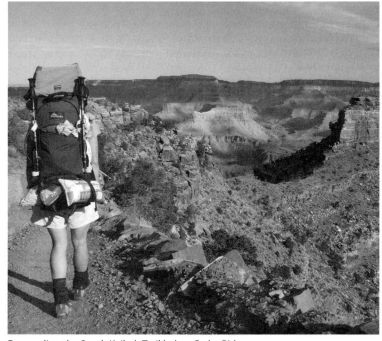

*Photo: Douglas Bock*

Descending the South Kaibab Trail below Cedar Ridge

# A Location Hike

Hiking is more than exercise—it is a time to be outdoors and therefore to absorb your surroundings. I am always a little disappointed to pass people so intent on reaching a destination or staring so closely at the bottoms of their hiking poles that they don't notice the flowers, the rocks, the birds, or the general landscape.

Hikes can be thought of as somewhere on a continuum from "destination hikes" to "location hikes." On a destination hike the sights along the way are overshadowed by those at the end point—many a summit hike or walk through forest to a spectacular lake fits into this category—and hikers are mostly forgiven for just trekking to the end. On a location hike, there is something new and spectacular to see every few steps down the trail, yet no single location that is universally judged "most beautiful." Hikes in the Grand Canyon are the ultimate location hikes, so plan an itinerary that gives you down time—be that many extra five-minute breaks to see what you pass or an extra day to give you more time to wander around.

## WHY YOU SHOULD BUY—AND CARRY—THIS BOOK

If you have ever searched for books on the Grand Canyon you were likely overwhelmed by the large number of generally excellent books written on its trails, natural history, human history, accidents, and more, leaving you wondering whether there's space for yet another title. If you wish to read individual books that delve into the region's botany, geology, prehistory, pioneer history, tourist attractions, on-trail hiking, or off-trail exploration, then the bibliography on page 164 suggests a healthy foundation for a Grand Canyon library. However, if you plan to visit the Grand Canyon infrequently (until its spirit captures you and you decide to return often), this book provides you an introduction to most of these topics, all focused on the two corridor trails descending from the South Rim: the Bright Angel and South Kaibab trails.

The primary goal of this book is to help you plan: how to get permits, what gear you should carry, how fast you should walk, what dangers you should avoid, and so on. However, it is also slim enough to tuck into your backpack for your journey to the river. Trail descriptions and maps aid you on your endeavor. In addition, ample human history and natural history sections inform you about topics from trail construction to commonly observed birds and plants. As you proceed first down to the Colorado River and then back up to the rim, you will take water, food, and rest breaks. As you sit in the shade on a hot summer day or enjoy a bit of midwinter warmth, pull out this book and learn about your surroundings.

## WHY YOU SHOULD NOT DAYHIKE

Grand Canyon National Park has a clear policy of telling people not to attempt to hike to the river and back in a day, and as a result, this book focuses on the information needed to complete an overnight trip to the Colorado River. When I first learned of the park's policy, it seemed quite extreme. I had not found the dayhike particularly taxing, and I have, on my trips to the canyon, met a lot of other hikers completing the hike in a single day without difficulty—granted these trips were in spring, fall, and winter, not midsummer. It seemed that a better approach would have been to emphasize attempting such a committing walk only during cooler months and emphasizing the need to start very early, be "slow and steady," and take sufficient breaks, especially during the heat of the day. Maybe they should instead instruct people to stay out of the Inner Gorge when midday temperatures exceed 85°F?

However, as rangers rattled off the number of rescues and fatalities suffered by people attempting a dayhike to the river, even in spring and fall, it became clear that a blanket recommendation was a pragmatic approach. Indeed, there are more deaths resulting from environmental conditions in May and June than in July and August, presumably because visitors don't appreciate how hot temperatures are during late spring, especially in the Inner Gorge where there is little shade during these near-solstice months. Many people do not know their physical limits and do not know when they are approaching their limit, leading to severe cases of hyponatremia and heatstroke (see page 54). Moreover, the enormous number of midsummer rescues endangers the lives of rescuers and costs the park—and the hikers being rescued—a lot. The information in this book is of course still accurate if you wish to dayhike, but I dissuade you from doing it.

*Inner Gorge refers to the steep gorge of Vishnu Schist and Zoroaster Granite below the Tonto Platform. Inner Canyon is anywhere below the canyon rim.*

Leaving national park policy aside, there are many more good reasons to take multiple days: Completing the hike as a dayhike accentuates the endurance aspects of the hike and takes away from the magic of the canyon and the natural history, because you have much less time to sit and absorb your surroundings. Plus you miss the beautiful morning and evening light from its depth. Many people probably attempt a dayhike because they did not reserve a wilderness permit. Others are people who do not enjoy the extra weight of an overnight pack or simply do not enjoy camping. If you fall into these categories, consider returning for a second trip when you have a backpacking reservation and can travel very light, when nighttime temperatures are warm or you have made a reservation to spend the night at Phantom Ranch.

# Human History

## NATIVE PEOPLES

The Colorado Plateau, although not the Grand Canyon, has been inhabited for at least 13,000 years, as evidenced by spearheads found in the region. The first of the southwestern Paleo-Indians, the Clovis culture, preferred the open plains areas to canyon country and are thought to have entered the Grand Canyon region rarely. More artifacts have been found from the ensuing Folsom culture, but their population densities on the Colorado Plateau would also have been low. The people of both cultures hunted the large mammal species that went extinct at the end of the ice age—possibly in part because of the hunting pressure. (It makes sense that these groups spent little time along the Colorado River. Can you imagine wooly mammoths and giant sloths descending into contorted canyons?)

The Archaic culture began by definition 8,500 years ago, and by 8,000 years ago people of this culture inhabited the Grand Canyon area. They too were a nomadic hunter-gatherer culture and had no permanent habitations. Over the subsequent six millennia, the distribution of people and especially their population densities fluctuated greatly, dictated largely by natural climatic fluctuations. During dry periods there were fewer predictable water sources and probably fewer game animals to hunt.

The descendants of the Archaic culture are the people of the Basketmaker culture, distinguished by the beautiful baskets they made. The Basketmaker culture began around A.D. 1, and by A.D. 500, at the latest, the people of this culture were farming corn, squash, and beans. This change in food source meant that the people were no longer nomadic, instead building more permanent habitations: pithouses as living quarters and shelters for food storage. However, even after they began to farm, the Basketmaker people living in the Grand Canyon continued to depend partially on wild game and wild plants. This flexibility gave them an advantage over tribes to the south that relied more heavily on farming; because of their use of wild food sources they maintained a more balanced—and healthier—diet than the tribes relying mostly on corn did.

Around A.D. 700 the Basketmaker culture transitioned to the Puebloan culture, designated by its aboveground rock and clay living quarters and its creation of ceramics. Pithouses were no longer used as houses, but in some regions, including the Grand Canyon, similar-shaped ceremonial kivas were central to the culture. The several centuries from A.D. 700 until A.D. 1140 were a period of cultural expansion and population growth across the Colorado Plateau and also a time of sufficient rainfall. The Puebloan villages from this era dot the entire Colorado Plateau—see page 161 for possible locations to visit after your Grand Canyon hike.

Particularly during the period from A.D. 1050 to A.D. 1100 settlements were established at many locations deep within the Grand Canyon. The small deltas that exist where side tributaries merge with the Colorado River were ideal for farming, including the mouth of Bright Angel Creek (see sidebar on page 7). River terraces, which are built up during periods of abundant runoff, were also used for farming. Many of the people had a second farm site on the canyon rim, allowing them to grow crops across more months of the year.

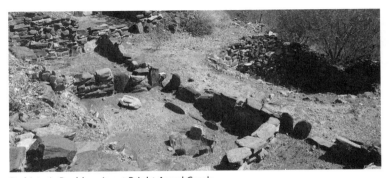

Prehistoric Pueblo ruins at Bright Angel Creek

Then, a 50-year drought from A.D. 1100 until A.D. 1150 coincided with a period of mass exodus from the Grand Canyon to the south. In the Grand Canyon an extended drought meant many springs dried up and the Colorado River terraces eroded. However, anthropologists do not believe that the climatic shift was solely responsible for their departure. The Kachina religion, practiced to the south, also enticed the Puebloan people southward. Despite the various pressures to move southward, some artifacts indicate a few Puebloans stayed in pockets of the Grand Canyon for many years after most people disappeared. (The Basketmakers and the Puebloan people are also known as the Anasazi, a frequently used term for the prehistoric people of the Colorado Plateau region. The Hopi, their descendants, prefer that this term not be used, as it is a derogatory Navajo term, meaning "enemy ancestor.")

A second group of people, the Cerbat/Pai, migrated from the Mojave Desert to the Grand Canyon region close to the time of the collapse of the Puebloan culture and settled the plateau country and fertile tributary valleys to the south of the Colorado River. The only Native Americans in the Grand Canyon region today are descendants of these people: the Havasupai tribe inhabiting Havasu Canyon to the west (downstream) of the corridor trails and the Hualapai tribe living on a reservation west of Grand Canyon National Park. While the tribes now live farther west, the Havasupai once farmed Indian Garden on the Bright Angel Trail.

The Southern Paiute also inhabited the Grand Canyon region for approximately six centuries until the arrival of white men, predominantly living on the north side of the Colorado River. The Paiute were not farmers; they lived solely on what they hunted and gathered.

## PUEBLO AT BRIGHT ANGEL CREEK

The ruins of a pueblo are visible at the mouth of Bright Angel Creek, between the Bright Angel Creek Campground and the mule bridge. The kiva was built when the site was first occupied, around A.D. 1050, while the living area dates to A.D. 1100. By A.D. 1140 this site, like most habitations along the Colorado River, was abandoned because of increasing drought. Major John Wesley Powell recorded this site during his first descent of the Colorado River.

## PIONEERS

The first view of the Grand Canyon by a nonnative person was in 1540 by a Spanish party led by Francisco Vasquez de Coronado. They were unimpressed with the difficult landscape, and Native Americans continued to be the only inhabitants of the area for many years. Only in 1826 did a party of fur trappers reach the rim; they were likewise disappointed by the steep, deep, contorted canyon and large river—and didn't recruit others to the location.

Explorers and settlers were first drawn to the area in larger numbers after Major John Wesley Powell explored the length of the

### MAJOR JOHN WESLEY POWELL

Because of his two pioneering descents down the Colorado River in 1869 and 1871, John Wesley Powell's name is synonymous with the Grand Canyon region. When he boarded the *Emma Dean*, a boat he had named after his wife, he was not new to river exploration. Already in 1856, at age 22, he had rowed a length of the Mississippi River, followed by the Ohio River the next year.

Powell grew up in the Midwest on a succession of farms, as his parents moved about. His strong interest in natural history emerged in 1857 while taking a botany course at Oberlin College in Ohio. In subsequent years he made extensive botanical and zoological collections across the Midwest, before changing his focus to geology. With the onset of the Civil War, he enrolled immediately in the Union Army and had risen to the rank of captain when he lost an arm at the Battle of Shiloh. After the Civil War he accepted a geology professorship at Wesleyan University. He was recognized as being an outstanding scientist—in particular one who had high standards and was very resourceful and endlessly inquisitive. This position allowed him to spend the summer of 1867 making scientific collections in what is now Colorado. In 1869 he returned west with the goal of exploring the virtually unmapped Green and Colorado rivers.

On May 24, 1869, his party of ten men departed Green River, Wyoming (not Green River, Utah), with ten months of provisions; six men exited at the mouth of the Colorado

Grand Canyon by boat in 1869 and 1871. He too discovered that the country was rough and dangerous, but viewed the difficulties as an adventure and the Grand Canyon as a place of scientific interest, rather than somewhere to avoid. Indeed, just two years after his first, rather disastrous trip, he returned to descend the river a second time and continue his scientific explorations. Following the 1871 excursion he began to promote the Grand Canyon as a tourist venue. However, it was initially the possibility of mineral riches that drew people, with hundreds arriving at the North Rim of the Grand Canyon in 1872 for a short-lived gold rush. No mineral riches were found in the vicinity of Bright Angel and South Kaibab trails,

River, near the confluence with the Virgin River more than three months later. They were nearly out of supplies, because of losses each time boats capsized. (One man left just days into the expedition, unnerved by the adventure. The other three exited the Grand Canyon near Separation Rapid, just two days before the end of the canyon and were likely killed by either Indians or Mormons as they made their way back to civilization.)

With the knowledge gained on this first expedition, he returned in 1871 with a new crew. Less drama pervaded this descent of the Colorado River, allowing important natural history collections to be made and much geologic information to be recorded.

The well-known Powell continued to make important scientific and "societal" contributions in the western U.S. He was involved in the creation of the U.S. Geological Survey, established to administer surveys like those he carried out in the Grand Canyon, and served as its second director from 1881 to 1894. He advocated against dividing the southwestern U.S. into the standard 160-acre homesteads, realizing that this approach was inappropriate for the region; much larger blocks of lands and boundaries along water divides were required. He realized as well that water was a limited resource that must be shared downstream. Also, unlike many others in this era, he greatly respected for the Native American tribes in the Southwest, studying their cultures and languages and petitioning the U.S. government to care better for them.

but many prospects and a few larger mines exist within the park, including the prominent Orphan Mine, a copper and then uranium mine that can be viewed at Powell Point, as well as a large copper vein along the Grandview Trail. A few small mine shafts exist along the Bright Angel Trail, both near the top of Devils Corkscrew and partway down Pipe Creek.

Tour guides and tourists soon displaced most of the miners. John Hance was the first true settler on the South Rim, arriving in 1883. A drifter drawn to the Grand Canyon's possible mineral riches, he quickly realized mining was not an efficient way to earn money and began guiding tourists to the Colorado River the following year. In subsequent years, the tourism business expanded rapidly, as more and more prospectors arrived on the South Rim and many realized that tourism was a more reliable source of income.

Among the miner-turned-tour-guides are Ralph Cameron, his brother Niles Cameron, and partner Pete Berry. In 1890 they obtained a mining claim at Indian Garden from the previous claimants. They quickly expanded the Havasupai route along the Bright Angel Fault into a trail, the predecessor of the contemporary Bright Angel Trail, and charged tourists a dollar to descend the trail. They soon constructed a tent camp at Indian Garden and Cameron's hotel on the rim followed in 1903. (See section on trail history and construction, page 13, for more information.)

The tourism business required more than tour guides, and many settlers found profitable niches. Among them, Ellsworth Kolb and his brother Emery began a South Rim photography business in 1902, building a studio, today's Kolb Studio, near the start of the Bright Angel Trail. They photographed parties descending the trail and then rushed to Indian Garden—the closest source of freshwater—to develop the photographs so that people could purchase prints on their return later than day.

Tourism was helped along by the fact that the Santa Fe Railway had completed tracks across northern Arizona in 1883, stopping in Williams just 65 miles from the South Rim and thereby providing relatively easy access for visitors from across the U.S. Before long, plans were in progress to build a spur line to the South Rim. William O'Neill, an early South Rim entrepreneur, organized funding and began to construct the route in 1897, laying tracks due south to meet the Santa Fe Railway's tracks in Williams. Following his death in 1898, the Santa Fe Railway purchased the tracks and constructed the last 10 miles of track to the canyon. Opened in 1901, it ferried visitors in comfort—especially once the railway company and concession partner, the Fred Harvey Company, constructed elegant hotels and restaurants on the canyon rim. The construction of the new road to the South Rim during the 1920s triggered the demise of the train service, and the railway ceased to run in 1968. In 1989, the historical route was resurrected and the historical depot in Williams refurbished.

## PHANTOM RANCH

Phantom Ranch is a collection of backcountry cabins, bunkhouses, and a dining hall located approximately one mile north of the mouth of Bright Angel Creek—a third of a mile upstream of the Bright Angel Creek Campground. The current structures were built beginning in 1922, designed by Mary Colter under contract with the Fred Harvey Company. She initially designed five buildings, but the resort was so popular that they built more structures. By 1930 the ranch appeared much as it does today. Only the hiker dorms were added much later.

The first structures at this location predate this. In 1903, Edwin "Dee" Woolley, a rancher from Kanab, Utah, and colleagues formed the Grand Canyon Transportation Company with the intent of building a cable across the Colorado River and a trail up to the North Rim via Bright Angel Creek, to be called the Grand Canyon Toll Road. They viewed a South Rim to North Rim trail system as the easiest way to increase tourism on the North Rim; to the north, the rail line stopped in Marysvale, approximately 200 miles north

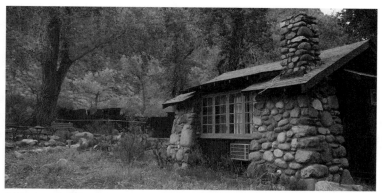

A Phantom Ranch cabin

of the North Rim. They decided upon Bright Angel Creek as the best corridor, for François Matthes, a surveyor and geologist, had already created a rudimentary trail in 1903. They viewed the lower reaches of Bright Angel Creek as a good place for a guesthouse.

Only slight progress was made until 1906 when David Rust, Woolley's son-in-law and a schoolteacher, took on the job of trail foreman. His journal indicates that the construction of the trail proceeded much as expected, but the construction of the cable involved much effort and numerous false starts. The first party finally crossed the Colorado River on September 20, 1907. In 1906, Rust and his crew also built the first dwellings at the Phantom Ranch site. They planted a garden, a small orchard, and many hundreds of cottonwood cuttings, obtained upstream from Phantom Creek, for shade. In subsequent summers they upgraded the accommodations and planted more trees in anticipation of a stream of wealthy guests. Unfortunately, relatively few tourists made use of this cross-canyon corridor, and although Rust continued to spend each summer until 1915 running his cable car and the Rust Camp, it never earned money for the Grand Canyon Transportation Company. In 1919 the newly founded national park took over possession of his cable car and trail.

## MARY COLTER

Mary Colter's name is inexorably linked with Grand Canyon architecture. She was first hired by the Fred Harvey Company to decorate Alvarado Hotel in Albuquerque in 1901. She began her work on the South Rim of the Grand Canyon in 1905, designing Hopi House. In subsequent years she designed Lookout Studio (1914), Hermit's Rest (1914), the Watchtower at Desert View (1932), Bright Angel Lodge (1935), and most relevant for a Grand Canyon hiker, Phantom Ranch in 1922. She designed her buildings to be in harmony with the natural surroundings, using local materials and architectural designs that caused the buildings to effectively merge with the landscape. Her buildings are beautiful exemplars of the style known as National Park Service rustic. At Phantom Ranch, for example, the cabins are built (mostly) of local rock, colored to blend with the surroundings, and spaced at irregular intervals.

## TRAIL HISTORY AND CONSTRUCTION

The Bright Angel Trail is a historic Indian trail used by people for millennia to access the inner canyon and the Colorado River. By the 1870s miners were entering the Grand Canyon and descending this same route. Ralph Cameron and his brother Niles acquired mining claims along the Bright Angel Trail in 1890. They quickly realized that the money was not in mining, but instead in tourism. They therefore took advantage of a law that allowed the "builders of a trail" to collect a toll for its use. In 1890 and 1891 they improved the Havasupai trail to Indian Garden and in 1898 completed a new trail down to the Colorado River. From 1903 until the 1920s they charged each person a dollar to descend the Bright Angel Toll Road (also called the Cameron Trail). These fees were introduced to keep money flowing their way once competing South Rim accommodations were constructed and disrupted their previous near-monopoly on housing Grand Canyon Village visitors.

The Santa Fe Railway and Fred Harvey Company, which ran the concessions associated with the railroad (and had built Phantom Ranch), the National Park Service, and other government agencies wished to invalidate Ralph Cameron's mining claims and take control of the trail that departed from the rapidly expanding Grand Canyon Village. Moreover, Ralph Cameron took poor care of "his" trail and the Indian Garden Campground. In 1913 the U.S. Forest Service sued Ralph Cameron over his unused claims, which led to a 1920 U.S. Supreme Court decision that dissolved his claims and turned the trail over to Coconino County. However, Cameron succeeded in continuing to collect tolls. He was also active in local politics and in 1924 convinced the citizens of Coconino County to vote against selling the Bright Angel Trail to the National Park Service.

To avoid requiring tourists to support the Cameron brothers, as soon as the Grand Canyon became a national park in 1919, the park service began arranging for the construction of an alternative route, which would become the South Kaibab Trail. They moved forward quickly following the November 1924 election and by December 1 of that year had $50,000 for the project, had ordered construction materials, and had amassed two 20-worker teams. One team would begin at the Colorado River and the other at Yaki Point. They had hoped to complete the trail by May, but it took until mid-June for the two teams to meet up because of the difficulty in blasting into solid rock and winter storms that delayed work. The final cost for the project was $73,000. The trail was dedicated on June 15, 1925. Except for the section of the trail below the Tipoff, the South Kaibab Trail did not follow an existing route.

The new trail was named for the Kaibab Plateau, a name suggested by J. R. Eakin, the first superintendent of Grand Canyon National Park. National Park Service Director Stephen Mather selected this name over other possibilities: Yaki Trail, indicating its descent from near Yaki Point and Phantom Trail, an option promoted by the Fred Harvey Company since the trail descends directly to their Phantom Ranch.

The National Park Service finally took control of the Bright Angel Trail in 1928, when Coconino County traded it in return for the park service funding a new road from Williams to Grand Canyon Village. The park service then reconstructed the Bright Angel Trail between 1929 and 1938; they decreased the grade of the trail, including the section above the 3-Mile Resthouse (1930–1931) and through the Devils Corkscrew (1929), built a trail alongside the wash upstream of Indian Garden (1930), routed the trail through the Tapeats Narrows (1929), and built a trail alongside Pipe Creek (1938). The trail had previously dropped down the Bright Angel Fault at nearly three times the grade it is today, simply followed the Garden Creek wash, diverted east of Garden Creek on the Tonto Platform, dropped down the Salt Creek Drainage (the seep you cross toward the top of Devils Corkscrew), and continued nearly straight down to Pipe Creek. The old, much steeper switchbacks can still be seen as you descend the Devils Corkscrew to Pipe Creek.

In addition to acquiring and retrofitting these important corridor trails, the park service lost no time in building a bridge across the Colorado River that was accessible to stock. In 1921 they completed a wooden suspension bridge to replace Rust's cable car. Unfortunately this bridge was susceptible to great contortions, even flipping over, and in 1928 a sturdier bridge, the current Kaibab Suspension Bridge (or "black" or "mule" bridge), was constructed. The eight 550-foot-long main suspension cables were each carried to the bottom of the canyon by a team of 42 Havasupai Indians.

The River Trail, the 1.7-mile trail along the Colorado River between the Bright Angel Trail and the Kaibab Suspension Bridge, was built between 1933 and 1936 by the Civilian Conservation Corps, under park service supervision. Long sections were blasted into vertical rock, providing hikers with airy views into the river. Until its con-

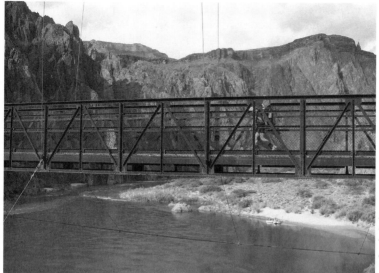

Photo: Douglas Bock

Crossing the Kaibab Bridge

struction, hikers descending the Bright Angel Trail and wishing to cross to the north side of the river, would leave the Bright Angel Trail just beyond Indian Garden and cross over on the trail that followed the Tonto Platform to the South Kaibab Trail. The last of the corridor trail network, the Silver Bridge was constructed in the 1960s as part of the transcanyon water system.

# Natural History

In many locations, people interested in natural history, which includes all information about the natural world, focus their attention on the plants and animals, and think of the geology as a backdrop. In the Grand Canyon the geologic features strike even the most ardent biologists. Not only is the geology visually grabbing, but also it is quickly apparent what a strong influence the geology, from rock type to topographic features, has on where plants and animals live. Consider for instance that different rock layers decompose to form soils with different nutrients and textures, affecting water-holding capacity and water availability, and therefore plant cover.

Even more apparent to a casual hiker, consider how variable the topography can be. For instance, some rock layers erode easily forming slopes, while others are cliffs, each creating unique habitats required and tolerated by different species. Where a north-facing cliff and gentler topography meet is a small patch of real estate that remains shadier and cooler, allowing a unique collection of species to establish. Rock formations with alternating layers of sandstone and shale, may create small platforms of soil underlain by fractured rock—if a tree takes root, it might find moister soil deep down. A wash that carries water occasionally will host different species than the dry terraces to either side. This variation in physical features creates patchiness in resources and in turn leads to a surprising diversity in plants and animals. As you explore the inner canyon, consider the interactions between the physical and biological worlds.

## GEOLOGY

Quite simply, the Grand Canyon is unbelievable because of its geologic features. As you stand at a vista point and peer into and across the canyon, you are marveling at the geology: staring at the exceptionally wide and deep canyon and the nearly horizontal layers of colorful rock. Generations of talented geologists have sought to understand what combination of geologic events created this landscape. Individuals with different geologic specialties have contemplated different aspects of the picture, weaving together their conclusions with the data collected by others to present a coherent story of the Grand Canyon's geologic history. However, the sleuthing continues—evidence to decipher some pieces of the story is simply missing. The story of the Grand Canyon presented today, in this book and at vistas throughout the park, may stand the test of time or may be quite different if you revisit the park in a generation.

Questions will probably leap to mind as you gaze at the canyon. You may wonder why such a deep canyon exists and how it formed. Or you may contemplate why there are so many different layers or rock, how they got there, and why some are flat, but others steep?

To answer these clusters of questions, and others, I describe the tectonic regimes to which the Grand Canyon area was subjected from 1.8 billion years ago until today, as the tectonic surroundings dictate many of the geologic processes that are recorded. These descriptions include information about the environments that led to the creation of the three main rock groups in the Grand

Canyon: the Grand Canyon Metamorphic Suite, the Grand Canyon Supergroup, and Paleozoic sedimentary layers. (See page 126 for descriptions of features that identify each rock layer.)

This brief description of the Grand Canyon's geology is obviously incomplete. If learning a few tidbits piques your curiosity to learn more about the past and present processes that have created the landscape, check out the numerous books written on Grand Canyon geology (see page 164). *Carving Grand Canyon* by Wayne Ranney is especially recommended both to learn about what forces combined to create the Grand Canyon and to understand how geologists use field evidence to discern geologic processes. *Ancient Landscapes of the Colorado Plateau*'s scope (by Ron Blakey and Wayne Ranney) is broader than the Grand Canyon, but it does a superb job of describing historical environments in the Grand Canyon region, both through narrative and maps. *Hiking the Grand Canyon's Geology* by Lon Abbott and Terri Cook provides a good introduction to the region's geology, detailed information on the formation of the many rock layers, and a geologic guide to take with you as you hike along either of the trails described in this book. The U.S. Geological Survey provides an online geologic map and annotated photos from the South Kaibab and Bright Angel trails at: http://3dparks.wr.usgs.gov/grca/index.html.

## CATEGORIZING ROCKS BASED ON ORIGIN

Geologists divide rocks into three categories. A **sedimentary rock** is formed either when mineral grains are transported to a site of deposition and subsequently cemented together or by chemical precipitation at the depositional site. An **igneous rock** is formed by the solidification of molten rock, or magma. Igneous rock that has solidified above the Earth's surface is termed volcanic and that below the Earth's surface is termed intrusive. A **metamorphic rock** forms when an existing rock is deformed because of high temperature or pressure, causing its mineral composition and/or texture to change. The Grand Canyon contains igneous and metamorphosed sedimentary and igneous rocks (in the Inner Gorge) and sedimentary rocks (the near-horizontal layers above the Inner Gorge).

### The tectonic regimes and resultant rocks

The nearly two-billion-year-old rock record at the Grand Canyon shows that a succession of different tectonic regimes occurred over time, which led to the formation of the three different rock groups that outcrop along the Bright Angel or South Kaibab trails. There were also periods of time when little occurred, rocks were being eroded away, or canyons carved.

**Collisions, 1.8 billion to 1.4 billion years ago:** About 1.8 billion years ago the location that would become the Grand Canyon was an oceanic basin that lay between the incipient North American Plate (to the northwest) and a volcanic island chain (the Yavapai Arc to the southeast). By 1.7 billion years ago the oceanic crust that carried the Yavapai Arc was being pushed over the edge of the North American Plate. In the process, the sediment in the intervening ocean basin was buried, twisted, heated, and hence metamorphosed to form the Vishnu, Brahma, and Rama schists, collectively known as the Grand Canyon Metamorphic Suite, or colloquially as the Vishnu Schist or basement rocks. Meanwhile, deeper sediments were completely melted. The resultant magma rose through cracks in the schist and cooled to form the intermingled Zoroaster Granite (and related rocks), a light-colored, often pinkish rock. Later, there

## PLATE TECTONICS

The surface of the Earth is composed of thin, rigid pieces termed plates. The 14 larger plates and many smaller microplates float and rotate slowly atop the more liquid inner layers of the Earth. Each of these plates is constantly moving—and in different directions from one another, so the plates collide, slide past one another, and pull away from one another, changing their position on the Earth's surface in the process. Colliding plates have created—and continue to create—the world's mountain ranges. In some cases, two plates move toward one another, the type of collision that created the European Alps. In other cases, one plate collides into and is shoved beneath a second plate, a process called subduction. Plates sliding past one another create large strike-slip faults like the San Andreas Fault in western California. Plates pulling apart create new and ever larger ocean basins, a process currently occurring in the Red Sea.

was a collision with a second volcanic island chain, the Mazatzal Arc. These collisions added much material to the edge of North America, moving its boundary well south of the Grand Canyon region.

**Little tectonic activity, 1.4 billion to 1.2 billion years ago:** Having the plate boundary south of the Grand Canyon set the stage for a long period of tectonic calm in the region. The mountain range that had formed from the collisions was slowly eroded, eventually allowing the deeply buried Vishnu Schist and Zoroaster Granite to rise to the surface. Some of their mass was eroded, flattening them by 1.2 billion years ago. The eroded surface is termed the Greatest Unconformity.

**Formation and existence of supercontinent Rodinia, 1.2 billion to 750 million years ago:** While the Grand Canyon was experiencing a period of tectonic calm and associated erosion, the global stage was being set for a set of massive collisions that formed the supercontinent Rodinia. Rodinia incorporated most of the Earth's land masses. Australia and Antarctica were welded onto the western edge of the North American continent, west of the Grand Canyon. Along the eastern edge of North America, the Grenville Orogeny, beginning 1.1 billion years ago, created the mountains of the eastern seaboard and apparently caused the western edge of North America to tip downward, creating a narrow sea at the border of North America and the Australian/Antarctic landmasses.

*When sedimentary rocks are horizontally layered, the layers indicate the order in which the sediment was deposited—the oldest sedimentary layer is at the bottom and the youngest on top.*

The Grand Canyon region was now a costal environment and the sediment that comprises the Grand Canyon Supergroup began to be deposited. Initially the shallow Bass Sea covered the area, depositing the calcareous sediment that constitutes the Bass Limestone. Subsequently, a decrease in water level led to the deposition of mud atop the limestone, creating the Hakatai Shale. Additional decrease in water level caused beach sands to be deposited, coalescing into the very erosion-resistant Shinumo Quartzite. What followed were small-scale encroachments and retreats of the sea, creating bedding shales and sandstones, the Dox Formation. The final formation in the first group of Supergroup rocks is the Cardenas Lava, dating to 1.1 billion years ago, coinciding with the Grenville Orogeny

## WHY ARE THERE SO MANY DIFFERENT TYPES OF SEDIMENTARY ROCK?

The type of sediment that is deposited is determined by a location's position on the landscape. Consider a shoreline environment: dunes along the coast (or farther inland) and beach sands become sandstones or quartzites (metamorphosed sandstones); mud and silt are deposited farther out to sea and become mudstones, siltstones, and shales; calcite accumulates in shallow tropical waters, both precipitating from the water and from the deposition of sea creatures. Fewer sediments are deposited and preserved in the interior of continents, which is why most sedimentary rocks are from shores, deltas, or shallow marine environments.

For different types of sediment to overlie each other, the shoreline's location must keep shifting. Many factors lead to never-ending movement in the position of the shoreline, including continuous variation in the strength of the sun's radiation and consequent changes in the amount of the Earth's water stored as ice. Over hundreds of thousands to millions of years, a single location will experience different sedimentary environments—a history preserved as consecutive layers of sedimentary rock.

and small-scale rifting in the Grand Canyon region. These first five formations are collectively known as the Unkar Group. The remaining Supergroup formations were deposited in the sea deep within Rodinia. Since they outcrop on neither the South Kaibab nor the Bright Angel trails, they are not described here.

**Breakup of supercontinent Rodinia, 750 million to 525 million years ago:** By 750 million years ago Rodinia was beginning to be pulled apart, as Antarctica and Australia headed westward. As the continents were separated, a series of large faults formed in the Grand Canyon region, including the Bright Angel Fault. These were normal faults, which form as a region is stretched and expanded, and result in some blocks of rock being dropped downward. The formation of these faults caused the Grand Canyon Supergroup strata to be tilted and blocks of Grand Canyon Supergroup rocks to be "dropped into" the basement rocks.

The period of breakup and faulting was also one of erosion and thousands of feet of sediment were removed from the landscape, including most of the Grand Canyon Supergroup strata and some depth of the basement rocks. These changes created the Great Unconformity, the boundary between the Grand Canyon Supergroup and the overlying Paleozoic sedimentary rocks.

Today the only Grand Canyon Supergroup strata that are preserved in the vicinity of the Bright Angel and South Kaibab trails are those on a down-dropped block below the Tipoff, termed Cremation *Graben* (German for "grave"). And even here, only the three lowermost strata, the Bass Limestone, Hakatai Shale, and Shinumo Quartzite are preserved.

## GEOLOGY DETERMINES WHERE THE TRAILS ARE LOCATED

If you visited vista points on the South Rim before embarking on your hike, you likely stared at the steep Kaibab Formation that forms a 350-foot-high cliff just about everywhere, providing few locations to descend below the rim. The Coconino Sandstone and Redwall Limestone form similarly impenetrable barriers. The Bright Angel Trail follows the Bright Angel Fault: Movement along the fault broke the solid rock, allowing erosion to proceed more rapidly. Eventually steep talus piles formed along the fault zone, allowing passage through otherwise vertical cliffs. In addition, the faulting has caused the rock on the southeast side of the fault to be about 200 feet lower than that on the northwest side, and the trail can snake back and forth across the fault depending on which side provides easier passage. The benefit of the fault scarp is especially visible where the Bright Angel Trail cuts through the Coconino Sandstone above the 1.5-Mile Resthouse and along Jacobs Ladder below the 3-Mile Resthouse. This fault first formed during the breakup of Rodinia 750 million years ago.

In contrast, the South Kaibab Trail is predominantly a ridge route that exploits locations where the normally steep rock layers have begun to erode, because they are outcropping along a narrow ridge. And here too, the passage through the Redwall Limestone follows a small fault.

**Passive margin, 525 million to 320 million years ago:** The breakup of Rodinia created a "passive margin," or tectonically quiet region, along the then western edge of North America, the Colorado Plateau region. Along such margins the seafloor often sinks rapidly continually creating more space for sediment to accumulate and allowing thick rock strata to form. The prominent striped layers in the Grand Canyon, a series of strata 4000 thousand feet thick, were deposited during this tectonic regime with the type of sediment changing with shoreline position and water depth. (Up to 18,000 feet of sediment was deposited on the Colorado Plateau, but only the lower strata are preserved in the Grand Canyon.)

The oldest (and lowest) of the layers is the **Tapeats Sandstone**, formed from former beach sands. The **Bright Angel Shale**, formed in shallow offshore waters, follows; the mud-sized particles comprising the shale were carried a short distance out to sea before being deposited. The **Muav Limestone**, the third layer, is constituted of a combination of calcite that precipitated and calcite-bearing shells that were deposited. Together, these three layers represent a 20-million-year period of rising sea level: While sand-sized sediment was amassing at one location, silt was being deposited in shallow water to the west, and calcite was accumulating even farther west. As the sea level rose, each environment shifted eastward, such that the three sediment types overlay each other in the Grand Canyon.

No records remain from the following 120 million years, probably because decreasing sea level at the end of this period allowed the upper sediment layers to erode. One intermediate layer, the **Temple Butte Limestone**, is present as a thick stratum in the western Grand Canyon, where waters were deeper, but along the Bright Angel and South Kaibab trails it exists only in eroded channels in the Muav Limestone. Note that each of the Grand Canyon's rock layers above the Muav Limestone is separated by an unconformity; some gaps in the rock record are brief, but others correspond to the removal of considerable sediment.

*When rock strata abutting one another do not represent a continuous time sequence, the surface between the two layers is referred to as an unconformity. This gap in time indicates that sediment was eroded from atop the lower stratum before the upper stratum was deposited.*

By 340 million years ago sea level was again rising, and much of the Colorado Plateau region was submerged beneath a large, shallow sea. Rivers transported little sediment to the region, creating the clear water environment that promoted the deposition of the thick layer known as the **Redwall Limestone**. The sea then retreated, eroding the top of this layer.

**Passive margin, but tectonic collisions to the east as Pangaea forms, 320 million to 250 million years ago:** Around 320 million years ago the supercontinent Pangaea, a landmass composed of all continents with North America along its western shore, began to form. The continental margin west of the Grand Canyon was still passive, but to the east, an ancestral mountain range, the Ancestral Rockies, rose. As this mountain range was uplifted, large quantities of sediment were eroded, first filling large basins immediately west of the mountain range, and later spilling westward to the Grand Canyon region. It was a desert environment all the way to the coast.

The **Supai Group** is composed of sediments from 320 to 285 million years ago. It is primarily red desert sands from the eroding mountains to the east. This sediment was deposited in an extensive coastal plain with enormous river deltas. During this time period Pangaea was centered over the South Pole and recurring glaciations (due to changes in sun strength) tied up vast quantities of water. As a result, sea level fluctuated more than 400 feet every 100,000 years, leading to repeated incursions of the sea, creating thin deposits of shale and limestone between the layers of desert sand.

The environment was similar when the next stratum, the **Hermit Formation**, was deposited, except that sea levels were lower and the formation is exclusively terrestrial. Large rivers continued to carry red mud and fine sand from the deserts to the east. As the continent became ever drier and the shoreline retreated farther west, large dunes spread across the Grand Canyon area. These giant sand dunes are preserved as the **Coconino Sandstone** (275 million years ago).

While the inland drought was continuing, the shoreline crept east again: By 273 million years ago, a very shallow sea again covered the area, leading to the deposition of intertidal deposits (the **Toroweap Formation**) and then deeper water where calcite accumulated (the **Kaibab Formation**; 265 million years ago). The Toroweap Formation contains gypsum and salt crystals, minerals formed by the evaporation of water.

*This marks the end of the sequence of sedimentation that is preserved today—the 4000-foot-thick sequence of multicolored strata that makes the Grand Canyon so spectacular.* However, the subsequent 250 million years are important as well: Those rocks needed to be lifted far above sea level and carved by flowing water. The remainder of the geologic description is therefore focused on the sequence of events that led to the creation of the Grand Canyon.

**Initial breakup of Pangaea, 250 million to 145 million years ago:** The Grand Canyon region was an arid terrestrial environment throughout this time. The 4000 feet of sediment, mostly desert sand, deposited atop the Paleozoic strata have since eroded. No sediments from this time period, the Mesozoic, survive in the Grand Canyon, but they are visible farther north on the Colorado Plateau.

**Subduction of the Pacific Plate begins, 145 million to 70 million years ago:** During this period, Pangaea continued to breakup, causing North America to be pushed westward, and the Pacific Plate to begin subducting beneath it. This new subduction zone created the beginnings of California's Sierra Nevada and thickened the continental crust west of the Grand Canyon, causing the Colorado Plateau to be depressed. An internal sea, the Mancos Sea, flooded the central parts of North America, including much of the Colorado Plateau. The water retreated toward the end of this period. *Around 70 million years ago, the strata that are now on the rim of the Grand Canyon were still at sea level.*

**Subduction expands eastward, 70 million to 18 million years ago:** Around 70 million years ago the effect of the subduction zone at the western edge of North America began to be felt much farther east, leading to rapid uplift inland. The uplift includes the Laramide Orogeny (the uplift of the Rocky Mountains), the formation of the Mogollon Highlands in southeastern Arizona, and the uplift of the Colorado Plateau. In the Grand Canyon, the outside pressures caused the buried rock strata to be uplifted, raising the rocks we see today far above sea level. *In order for the Colorado River to later carve such a deep canyon, the strata needed to be elevated; an ocean-bound stream can, after all, only carve down to sea level.* The strata were also compressed, leading to the formation of the East Kaibab Monocline, the arching of the rock layers into an elongate dome in the central Grand Canyon region. This episode of uplift was completed by 40 million years ago.

The Colorado Plateau, although raised far above sea level, remained lower than the surrounding mountain ranges. During this period, rivers in the Grand Canyon region flowed to the northeast, as sediment and water were transported out of the Mogollon Highlands, into giant lakes in northern Arizona and Utah. This drainage pattern persisted until at least 30 million years ago and possibly as recently as 18 million years ago.

Sometime between 30 and 18 million years ago drainage patterns may have begun to change, but very few details are known. The Colorado River system did not exist. Some water may have drained southward, but most stream systems still headed north. Much water may have drained into internal basins that did not connect to the ocean.

## WHY ARE THE RIMS DIFFERENT ELEVATIONS—AND DOES IT MATTER?

Both the South Rim and North Rim sit atop the Kaibab Formation. Although the layers appear flat from either vantage point, they are slightly slanted, and the North Rim is approximately 1000 feet higher than the South Rim, for these layers are bent into a broad arch, the East Kaibab Monocline. The apex of the arch is 12 miles north of the North Rim. The southern side of the arch slants gently downward from that point and drops 1000 feet between the North and South rims.

This difference in elevation has other implications: The angle of the rock layers means that water falling on the rims flows away from the South Rim, but is funneled toward the North Rim. Therefore, relatively little water flows down creeks from the South Rim, but considerable amounts flow down drainages beginning on the North Rim. As a result, less side-stream erosion has occurred on the south side of the canyon and the descent from the canyon rim to the Colorado River is much shorter and steeper than from the North Rim. The landscape is accordingly less complex; there are far more buttes and intricate side canyons on the north side of the river.

**Extension to the west, 18 million to 6 million years ago:** During this time period, stretching and thinning of western North America caused the Basin and Range Province in Nevada to form and the land surrounding the Colorado Plateau to decrease in elevation. Once the regions to the south and west were lower than the plateau, runoff began to etch south-flowing drainages, the direction of today's Colorado River.

However, sediment deposits suggest that the Colorado River itself did not exist until approximately 6 million years ago. Instead, there were still large inland lakes and shorter waterways that were not connected. Water likely flowed along some of the Colorado River's present path and through some of its major tributaries, although possibly opposite from the direction it does today. For instance, water may have flowed down the Little Colorado and then *up* Marble Canyon, but not through the main Inner Gorge of the Grand Canyon to the west of the confluence of these two drainages.

What caused these many rivers to coalesce into a single large drainage system is not definitively known, but two theories rise to the forefront. One is that the inland lakes suddenly joined together, possibly because of a catastrophic overflow of one of them, providing the force to cut through topographic barriers and integrate previously disconnected drainage systems. A second theory is headward erosion, whereby erosion causes waterways to move progressively upstream, cutting into slopes. Eventually this process destroys a ridge that had previously divided two drainages and connects the two stream systems. A combination of these two processes likely integrated the Colorado River system.

The final big event required for the creation of the modern Colorado River course is the creation of the Gulf of California, which occurred about 6 million years ago, and provided the Colorado River's outlet to the ocean.

**Glaciations and fault movements, 6 million years ago to present:** By 6 million years ago, the Colorado River followed its current course to the Gulf of California. Events during the past 2 million years contributed to significant downward erosion, allowing the canyon to achieve its depth. First, the past 2 million years have been a time of recurring glaciations and at the end of each glacial cycle, greatly increased runoff from the Rocky Mountains would have resulted in giant floods with enormous erosive power.

Second, the Colorado River is crosscut by multiple faults, where the side of the fault that descends coincides with the downhill side of the river. Each time the fault moved, the downhill side of streambed would suddenly have been lowered, creating a step termed a *knickpoint*. A river's erosive power slowly moves knickpoints upstream, in the process deepening the riverbed.

A second geologic event also created large and probably temporary knickpoints: There were large lava flows that dammed the Colorado River approximately 640,000 years ago. Although probably short-lived, these dams would have allowed enormous reservoirs to form along the Colorado River's course. When the dams broke or were eroded upstream, the water stored behind the dam would have been instantaneously released, providing massive erosive force.

## AN EVOLUTIONARY STORY

The physical conditions that create the rock strata you traverse are repeated again and again, creating multiple layers of limestone, shale, or sandstone. However, the Grand Canyon's sedimentary strata were deposited over 500 million years, and the fossils in successive strata record much of the evolutionary history of life.

At the time the Bass Limestone was deposited, the only lifeform was single-celled colonial bacteria called stromatolites, visible in the rock as wavy bands. Multicellular, shell-bearing, aquatic animals evolved by the start of the Cambrian era, 542 million years ago; the Bright Angel Shale contains abundant trilobites, an early shell-bearing creature. Worm burrows, termed *trace fossils,* are also abundant. By the time the Redwall Limestone was deposited, different invertebrates dominated the seas, and crinoids (a stalklike relative of starfish) and brachiopods are abundant in this layer. Unlike at the time of the Bright Angel Shale's deposition, plants and animals now colonized the land. Along the South Kaibab Trail, plant fossils are visible in the Hermit Formation; some specimens of ferns are on display on the west side of Cedar Ridge for all to observe. The Coconino Sandstone preserves reptile footprints. Stop and consider that these critters didn't exist when you are just a couple of miles farther down the trail.

## VEGETATION

Most hikers will consider their walk from the Grand Canyon's rim to the Colorado River—and back up again—to be simply "desert." Spring, summer, and fall temperatures are hot, the humidity is low, and the vegetation is sparse and prickly. However, you will in fact pass through four vegetation zones, each existing due to a specific combination of elevation, moisture availability, and temperature and each dominated by specific species. They are:

**Pinyon-juniper woodland:** Pinyon pine and juniper are the dominant species in this widespread southwestern plant community. At the Grand Canyon, this community exists on the South Rim and inside the canyon down to the Redwall Limestone. Ecologically, it demarcates the elevation that receives significant snow during the winter months. (For the first 1000 feet below the rim on the Bright Angel Trail, this community is interspersed with the mountain scrub and chaparral community, composed of species including Gambel oak, fernbush, serviceberry, and snowberry.)

**Blackbrush scrub:** This community is defined by the dominance of blackbrush and covers the Tonto Platform. Unless you head toward Plateau Point, the characteristic monostands of blackbrush are not observed along the Bright Angel Trail, since the trail descends along the Garden Creek drainage, first down the dry wash below Jacobs Ladder and then through riparian (streamside) vegetation below Indian Garden. On the South Kaibab Trail, you are in blackbrush scrub as you cross the Tonto Platform and approach the Tipoff.

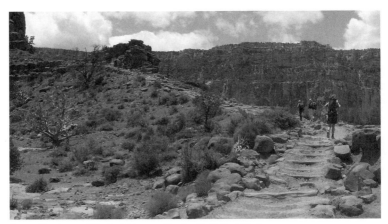

Ascending toward Cedar Ridge on the South Kaibab Trail

**Mojave Desert scrub:** This community exists below the Tonto Platform down to the Colorado River. The species growing here can withstand extremely high summer temperatures and many require milder winters. Although it is informally termed Mojave Desert scrub, the plant community contains many species not present in the Mojave Desert of southeastern California. For instance, species such as brittlebush and catclaw acacia that are typical of the warmer Sonoran Desert of southern Arizona exist in the Inner Gorge. Farther downstream, species such as honey mesquite, characteristic of the Chihuahuan Desert, enter the mix. Indeed, along the Colorado River corridor a unique combination of species grow, for three of North America's four deserts merge in this region.

**Riparian:** This community exists only in locations with permanent water, such as along the banks of the Colorado River and its side canyons. The availability of water means that large trees and dense thickets of shrubs and herbs are able to grow in these locations. The dominant species include Fremont cottonwood, coyote willow, seepwillow, saltcedar, honey mesquite, and catclaw acacia. The riparian vegetation along the Colorado River has changed significantly since the completion of the Glen Canyon Dam in 1964; water flows are now restricted and the river no longer floods as severely, a process that once scoured the vegetation along the banks and deposited vast quantities of sediment. Beginning in 1996 the Bureau of Reclamation has three times released higher flows from Glen Canyon Dam to replicate historic flooding. The largest flow occurred in March 2008, when they released twice the usual flow of water. Preliminary research indicates that this flood effectively mimicked natural floods, creating large sandbanks, reducing the establishment of nonnative plants, and creating backwater environments.

These vegetation zones can be identified by just a few dominant shrubs and trees, but more than 900 species occur below the canyon rims and in spring a diligent botanist might locate several hundred species along this walk. Any attentive hiker will notice many tens of distinctive and, when flowering, colorful species. Such diversity exists because the landscape is complex, creating many unique combinations of physical, chemical, and biological conditions. Each species prefers a certain soil depth, soil made from a specific rock, a specific small-scale climate, and a specific topographic position. Your walk will take you past geographic features that include solid rock, washes, steep slopes, seeps, small dunes, river terraces, the

## DESERT ADAPTATIONS

Colorful flowers attract your attention—and that of pollinators—but stare also at the leaves and stems of plants, for they you will remind you what life is like for plants in the region. For instance, shrubs and perennial herbs that grow in a desert environment must have traits that minimize water loss: Lack of leaves (e.g., cactus), drought-deciduous leaves (leaves that fall off in summer; e.g., blackbrush), small leaves (e.g., Mormon tea) and hairy leaves (e.g., brittlebush and big sagebrush) are all common desert adaptations. Most water loss occurs because plants need to cool their leaves by transpiring (evaporating) water, a process much like humans sweating. Minimizing leaf area and having leaf hairs to reflect light and keep leaves cooler are two very effective ways to preserve water.

However, plants require leaves, or at least green surfaces; the green color indicates plant parts that can photosynthesize, or turn the sun's energy into the sugars necessary for the plants to grow. In many species green stems compensate for limited leaf area. Drought-deciduous shrubs and many perennial herbs sprout leaves in spring when water is available and effectively hibernate during the hot summers. Other species are annuals. These plants grow for only a single season, germinating when soils are sufficiently moist and producing flowers and seeds in quick succession to avoid dry soils.

Tonto Platform, stream banks, ridges, and valleys, each home to a different collection of species.

Below are descriptions of 38 species along the Bright Angel and South Kaibab trails, including the most common species, as well as some showy, difficult-to-miss species that occur along a specific stretch of trail. They are organized by growth form (trees and larger shrubs, herbs and small shrubs, and cacti and agaves) and are approximately in order of their appearance from the canyon rim to bottom. A list of all species in the Grand Canyon is available on the Southwest Environmental Information Network: http://swbiodiversity.org/seinet/checklists/checklist.php?cl=94.

### Trees and Larger Shrubs

Shrubs are distinguished from trees by the number of branches that emerge from the soil surface: Trees have a single trunk, while shrubs have multiple trunks (or branches). For some species, local conditions determine which growth form individuals will display.

**Douglas fir *(Pseudotsuga menziesii)*:** Near the top of the Bright Angel Trail, these tall conifers grow in shaded, moister draws and right at the base of the wall of Coconino Sandstone. These cooler locations are the only place these tall conifers can survive at this elevation. Their needles attach singly to branches and their 2- to 3-inch cones are identified by the "rat tails" that emerge beneath each scale. *(pinyon-juniper woodland)*

**Utah juniper *(Juniperus osteosperma)*:** The Utah juniper and Colorado pinyon pine (see below) are the dominant species along the South Rim. These junipers, which can reach 20 feet in height, can be observed along both trails down to an elevation of approximately 5000 feet, although they are most abundant on the uppermost miles of the South Kaibab Trail. As with all junipers they have aromatic awl-like leaves, small blue berries, and reddish, shredding bark. *(pinyon-juniper woodland)*

**Colorado pinyon pine *(Pinus edulis)*:** Together with the Utah juniper, this pine tree is the dominant species in the pinyon juniper scrubland that dominates the South Rim and extends a little below Cedar Ridge on the South Kaibab Trail and around the 3-Mile Resthouse on the Bright Angel Trail. The edible nuts of the pinyon pine were an important food source for the Native American tribes inhabiting the Colorado Plateau and Great Basin. This often-shrubby species usually reaches a height of 15 to 20 feet and is identified by stiff needles that attach to branches in clusters of two. *(pinyon-juniper woodland)*

**Gambel oak *(Quercus gambelii)*:** The Gambel oak, which grows at elevations as low as 4000 feet, is along the first mile of the South Kaibab Trail and along the Bright Angel Trail above 3-Mile Resthouse. A shrub to a small tree, its leaves have rounded lobes, the classic oak leaf shape, and are winter deciduous. In fall the trees are covered with acorns. *(pinyon-juniper woodland)*

**Mexican cliffrose *(Purshia mexicana)*:** This large shrub, a relative of Apache plume (see below), is a common species from the canyon rim down to the Tonto Platform. You are especially likely to notice it on the upper portions of the Bright Angel Trail when it is covered with flowers during spring and possibly again in summer after a heavy monsoon. A member of the rose family, the five cream-colored petals are rose-shaped, just much smaller. The small leathery leaves are deeply dissected. During summer and fall, five long, featherlike tails emerge from the ends of the small, single-seeded fruit and decorate the plants. *(pinyon-juniper woodland* and *blackbrush scrub)*

**Apache plume *(Fallugia paradoxa)*:** These shrubs are difficult to miss as you ascend the shallow wash upstream of Indian Garden. By late spring, their white five-petal flowers give way to dense heads of more than 20 seedlike fruits, each with a wispy reddish tail. They are common throughout the canyon, especially in dry washes and along the outer (drier) edge of riparian corridors. *(blackbrush scrub* and *Mojave desert scrub)*

**Western redbud *(Cercis occidentalis)*:** In the Grand Canyon, western redbud grows both in well-watered locations and along dry washes. On these trails it is abundant in the Garden Creek riparian corridor and also along the west bank of the dry wash above Indian Garden. If you are hiking in early spring, it is difficult to miss, as the trees are covered with pink flowers. During the midseason months the tree can be identified by its round heart-shaped, smooth, glossy leaves, which turn brilliant colors in fall. *(riparian)*

**Fremont cottonwood *(Populus fremontii)*:** This tree with a tall, unbranched trunk is common along tributary streams, including at Indian Garden and along sections of Bright Angel Creek. Its broad, spade-shaped, deciduous leaves provide an excellent source of shade. Early settler David Rust planted the first cuttings at the Bright Angel Campground and Phantom Ranch; today new saplings are added (and watered) when floods destroy older trees. *(riparian)*

**Catclaw acacia *(Acacia greggii)*:** Catclaw acacia grows on dry slopes and in riparian areas, including dry washes, where it can form dense thickets. You will see it up to an elevation of 4800 feet in locations such as the bottom switchbacks on the South Kaibab Trail, the River Trail, and the Bright Angel Trail along Pipe Creek. This shrub (or tree) is named for the sharp, curved thorns that dot its branches. Like most acacias, its leaves are pinnately compound, meaning each "leaf" is composed of a long row of small "leaflets." Catclaw acacia's leaves are twice compound: there are 2 to 3 pairs of primary leaflets,

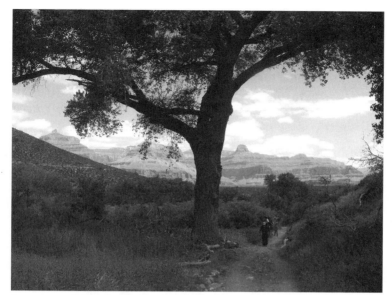

A cottonwood along Garden Creek on the Bright Angel Trail

each of which is a long stalk bearing up to 10 pairs of secondary leaflets. Its cream to light-yellow flowers grow in dense clusters resembling a duster. *(Mojave desert scrub* and *riparian)*

**Western honey mesquite *(Prosopis glandulosa)*:** Mesquite is often confused with catclaw acacia, since both are large shrubs with "pea pods" and pinnate leaves. However, a few characteristics readily differentiate them: mesquite, unlike catclaw acacia, has straight thorns and twice compound leaves with one pair of primary leaflets and 7 to 17 pairs of secondary leaflets. Rarely found along the section of the Colorado River you will walk, mesquite exists in Pipe Creek and along Bright Angel Creek around Phantom Ranch. Because of its deep roots, mesquite can grow along the dry outer reaches of riparian areas, but it does not establish within the flood zone. *(Mojave desert scrub* and *riparian)*

**Saltcedar *(Tamarix chinensis)*:** The saltcedar, or tamarisk, is an invasive species native to the Middle East. It has damaged many southwestern riparian areas, as it has deeper roots than native species, lowering the water table below the native species' roots—it is, however, very striking when covered in small light pink flowers. It currently grows along Pipe Creek, but the park service is trying to eradicate it. *(riparian)*

**Seepwillow or mule fat** *(Baccharis salicifolia)*: At the Bright Angel Campground, this species is abundant along the banks of Bright Angel Creek. Although its name refers to its narrow leaves that resemble those of a willow, it is actually a member of the sunflower family. And unlike those of the co-occurring coyote willow (see below) its leaves are coarsely toothed. Clusters of the white button-like flowers grow at the ends of branches and can be present much of the year. *(riparian)*

**Coyote willow** *(Salix exigua)*: This willow species is common along any Colorado River tributaries that flood regularly, including Bright Angel Creek. It has extremely narrow, untoothed leaves whose undersides are covered with fine hairs. As with all willows, they bear flowers in fluffy catkins. *(riparian)*

### Herbs and Small Shrubs

Herbs are annual and perennial species lacking woody stems. The shrubs included in this section have woody stems, but are similar in height to the herbs described. Most species described here are perennials, as they will be more predictably found at a given location. Most annuals and perennials flower in spring, when temperatures are warm, days are long, and soils are moist from winter rain and snow. Following a heavy monsoon, some annuals germinate a second time and some perennials bloom again.

**Common paintbrush** *(Castilleja applegatei ssp. martinii)*: This most common of the many paintbrush species in the canyon appears from the canyon rims down to the Colorado River corridor. True to their name, the flowers appear to have been dipped in paint, for the outer tips of the leaves surrounding the flower are brightly colored; the hidden flower petals are white to green. The paintbrush flowers are densely arranged around the flowering stalk, giving the appearance of a brush. All paintbrushes are hemiparasites, meaning they obtain some of their nutrients from nearby species through their roots; their roots grow intertwined with those of other species, especially certain grasses. *(pinyon-juniper woodland, blackbrush scrub, and Mojave desert scrub)*

**Smallflower globemallow** *(Sphaeralcea parvifolia)*: Along the Bright Angel trail, smallflower globemallow is common from the South Rim until near Indian Garden. It is likewise common along the upper stretches of the South Kaibab Trail. The salmon-orange flowers grow in long spikes, and new buds continue to open at the top of the flowering stalks through much of the year. The broad, slightly lobed leaves are covered with coarse hairs. Several closely related species in the region differ in features such as leaf shape and flower size; various species occur along the entire trail. *(pinyon-juniper woodland)*

**Southern mountain phlox** *(Phlox austromontana)*: This low-growing sub-shrub inhabits the upper miles of the Bright Angel and South Kaibab trails. Growing no more than 10 inches in height, the stems are densely covered with narrow, sharply pointed leaves. Light-pink flowers cover the plant in spring. The bottoms of the five petals are fused into a tube, while their tips splay open into a flat surface. *(pinyon-juniper woodland)*

**Eaton's firecracker** *(Penstemon eatonii)*: Of the many species of red penstemon (or beardtongue) in the park, Eaton's firecracker is one that you might see along rocky, dry sections of the upper reaches of both trails. All penstemon have long floral tubes, formed by five fused petals. In this species, the tube extends nearly to the ends of the petals, contrasting with other species where longer petal lobes extend beyond the tube. Their long, narrow leaves are attached to the stem in pairs. *(pinyon-juniper woodland)*

**Thickleaf penstemon** *(Penstemon pachyphyllus)*: This purple to periwinkle penstemon is common both on the South Rim and in rocky areas along the upper stretches of the Bright Angel and South Kaibab trails. The mouth of the flower tube is relatively broad, and the tips of the five petals are splayed open. As with many other penstemon, the flowers are arranged in circles along an elongate flowering head. *(pinyon-juniper woodland)*

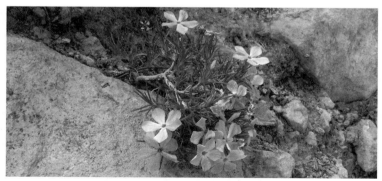

Southern mountain phlox

**Desert purple sage *(Salvia dorrii)*:** Present on both trails, this small shrub is especially prevalent on the South Kaibab Trail a little below Cedar Ridge. A low-growing, spreading shrub, it has small, ovate, gray-green, strongly aromatic leaves. Small purple, tubular flowers encircle elongate flowering stalks during the spring months. Unlike the ubiquitous sagebrush, desert purple sage is a relative of the culinary sages. *(pinyon-juniper woodland)*

**Green Mormon tea *(Ephedra viridis)*:** This species of Mormon tea is present along both trails until you drop below the Tonto Platform. It is an evolutionarily unusual species that might be a relative of the conifers (including pines and junipers). At first glance it appears to be a collection of stiff, green branches, earning the family the common name of "joint fir." However, if you look closely at the shrub, you can see small scalelike leaves growing from the stems. There are separate male and female individuals, with female plants producing larger seed-containing cones. In the Inner Gorge, it is replaced by other species of Mormon tea; the different species have, among other characteristics, different stalk colors and different branching patterns, most obvious if you can observe two species side by side. *(pinyon-juniper woodland* and *blackbrush scrub)*

**Big sagebrush *(Artemisia tridentata)*:** The big sagebrush grows above 5000 feet in elevation in the Grand Canyon and you will find it along both trails. The leaves of this shrub are wedge-shaped with three teeth at their broader end. They are also densely covered with hairs, giving them a grayish-green color. Its small disclike, yellowish flowers appear in late summer. *But don't be tempted to flavor your food with its aromatic leaves—this species is not a culinary sage! (pinyon-juniper woodland* and *blackbrush scrub)*

**Prickly poppy *(Argemone munita)*:** The large flowers of the prickly poppy, one of two closely related species that inhabit this region of the Grand Canyon, greet you along the Bright Angel Trail before you begin the climb up Jacobs Ladder. The other, the Roaring Spring prickly poppy, is present only along the North Kaibab Trail. Both species have five white petals that resemble crepe paper and surround a bright yellow center, composed of many stamens covered with yellow pollen. Their leaves live up to the flower's name—they are incredibly prickly. *(pinyon-juniper woodland* and *blackbrush scrub)*

**Colorado four o'clock *(Mirabilis multiflora)*:** It is impossible to miss the large cup-shaped magenta flowers of this sprawling species—if you reach the area just above Indian Garden by early morning. The four o'clock's name comes from when the flowers open: around 4 P.M., remaining open overnight to be pollinated by hawk moths and closing before the heat of the day. The repeatedly forked stems of this plant crawl along the ground, much like the related trailing four o'clock, but the Colorado four o'clock's flowers are larger (the tubes are 2 inches long) and the petals are not notched. *(pinyon-juniper woodland* and *blackbrush scrub)*

**Prince's plum *(Stanleya pinnata)*:** Following a wet winter, this relative of mustards lives up to its name. Yellow flowers cluster along the length of up to 6-foot-tall stems. Before long these develop into long seedpods, dangling from the flowering stalk like airy feathers. Its deeply lobed leaves are mainly clustered at ground level, with fewer along the stem. It prefers open slopes and is common on the Tonto Platform and, on the South Kaibab Trail, on the open slopes below Cedar Ridge. *(pinyon-juniper woodland* and *blackbrush scrub)*

**Desert trumpet *(Eriogonum inflatum)*:** Desert trumpet, a type of buckwheat, is as striking dead as alive. Its hollow stems are inflated into a large bulge below each branching point. Clusters of very small yellow flowers appear in summer (and sometimes spring). The stems remain standing unless strong winds or heavy snow disturb them; they can dot the landscape into the winter. Along the Bright Angel Trail they are especially common in the wash between Indian Garden and Jacobs Ladder, but occur along both trails down to river level. *(blackbrush scrub* and *Mojave desert scrub)*

**Blackbrush *(Coleogyne ramosissima)*:** Blackbrush, also known as burrobrush, is the dominant, and in places, only, species along the Tonto Platform. This shrub's name derives from its dark bark, which turns nearly black when wet. Blackbrush flowers lack true petals, but the four sepals—the leaflike structures that usually surround a flower bud—are yellow and showy. Its small, narrow dark green leaves are rolled under at the margins and attach to the thorn-tipped stems in clusters; its dense network of branches forms a thicket. It sheds its leaves during the summer. *(blackbrush scrub)*

**Mojave aster *(Xylorhiza tortifolia)*:** On the Bright Angel Trail, the Mojave aster is common from the bottom of Jacobs Ladder until you reach Pipe Creek. It is similarly common at mid-elevations on the South Kaibab Trail. In spring, the branches of this small shrub are covered with large, light purple daisylike flowers. Later in the year it is difficult to identify unless you are familiar with its narrow, distinctly toothed leaves. *(Mojave desert scrub)*

**Twining snapdragon** *(Maurandya antirrhiniflora)*: This trailing vine is found throughout the Inner Gorge and is especially prevalent along the lower half of the Devils Corkscrew and Pipe Creek. The tiny, bright pink flowers are shaped like those of a snapdragon and the leaves are arrow-shaped. *(Mojave desert scrub)*

**Yellow columbine** *(Aquilegia chrysantha)*: Like most columbines, this species requires much moisture, and grows only at seeps, at springs, and beside waterfalls. Along these trails, you will see it only at the spring just before you climb above Pipe Creek (on the Bright Angel Trail). At this location it grows en masse, and in spring can color the rock walls yellow. Each of the columbine's five petals forms a long backward-pointing spur. *(riparian)*

**Sacred datura** *(Datura meteloides)*: Sacred datura is common along Pipe Creek, the River Trail, and the lower stretches of the South Kaibab Trail. The large tubular white flowers are very poisonous and are the cause of at least one Grand Canyon fatality. (The 20-year-old victim sought the hallucinogenic effects of the plant by drinking a self-concocted datura tea. A day later, still high and incoherent, he attempted to cross the Colorado River and drowned.) Their shape and color are characteristic of a moth-pollinated species, and indeed they open in the late afternoon, bloom all night, and fade to a purplish hue by morning. *(Mojave desert scrub)*

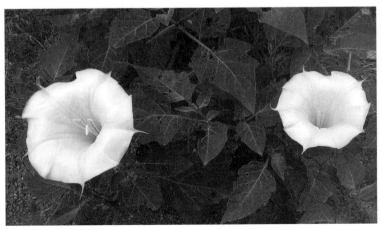

Sacred datura

**Brittlebush** *(Encelia farinosa)*: Of the several brittlebush species you will pass on your walk, this one is the most common in the Inner Gorge, but grows only to an elevation of about 3000 feet. Given sufficient rainfall, this shrub will be covered with bright yellow flowers resembling sunflowers throughout the spring. Its grayish-green leaves are densely covered in fine hairs to reflect sunlight and keep leaf temperatures cooler. *(Mojave desert scrub)*

**Rocknettle** *(Eucnide urens)*: Rocknettle grows in the rocky sections of the River Trail and at lower elevations along the South Kaibab and Bright Angel trails. The five petals splay open at the top of the tubular white flowers. Although not related to nettles, the long hairs on this species' buds and stems are reminiscent of its namesake. The margins of its round, dark green leaves are toothed. *(Mojave desert scrub)*

**Sand verbena** *(Abronia elliptica)*: You will see this species while crossing the short stretch of sand dunes along the River Trail. A trailing plant, its small tubular white flowers are arranged into a large sphere and its leaves are small, oval-shaped, and quite thick. *(Mojave desert scrub)*

### Cacti and Agaves

Cacti and agaves are not closely related species but are often grouped together in guidebooks due to their similarly prickly appearance.

**Century plant** *(Agave utahensis)*: Although most abundant on the Tonto Platform and the platform by Skeleton Point, the century plant grows from the canyon rim down to the Colorado River. When not in flower, the plant is a cluster of spine-tipped, sharptoothed succulent leaves. Large numbers of individual plants flower in wet years by rapidly sending up a very tall stalk covered with small yellow flowers. While some individuals die after flowering, others send up clones from underground stems, continuing the parent plant's genetic legacy. *(pinyon-juniper woodland, blackbrush scrub, and Mojave desert scrub)*

**Banana yucca** *(Yucca bacata)*: The banana yucca grows all the way to the South Rim, but is most obvious along the Tonto Platform. Like the century plant, it has a cluster of stiff spine-tipped leaves emanating from a central point. Its leaves have a white margin that peels into picturesque curlicues. In spring, a shoot, which does not extend far beyond the leaf tips, appears from the center of the plant, with large, drooping white flowers opening in April and May. *(pinyon-juniper woodland* and *blackbrush scrub)*

**Claret-cup cactus** *(Echinocereus triglochidiatus)*: The claret-cup cactus forms a cluster of cylindrical, ribbed stems, each about 4 inches in diameter. The bright white spines stick straight out from the stems. And this is a species that is impossible to miss when in bloom: The 2- to 4-inch-long flowers are a vibrant red, and unlike most other cacti, its petals are rounded. It grows from canyon rim to the river, but you will see most individuals at the lower elevations. *(blackbrush scrub* and *Mojave desert scrub)*

**Grizzly bear cactus** *(Opuntia erinacea)*: From a distance, the grizzly bear cactus has a grayish appearance—its broad, flat blades are very densely covered with flexible spines, some up to 4 inches long. Its magenta or yellow flowers closely resemble those of related species, such as the beavertail and desert prickly pear cacti. This species is common on the Tonto Platform. *(blackbrush scrub* and *Mojave desert scrub)*

**Engelmann prickly pear cactus** *(Opuntia engelmannii)*: This species of cactus forms a dense barrier on either side of the trail as

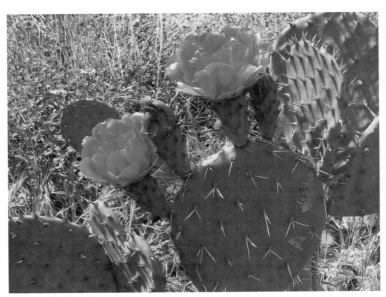

Engelmann prickly pear cactus

you pass the ranger station at Indian Garden. In late spring when it is in bloom, you are greeted by a beautiful display of large yellow or magenta flowers—each individual has a single flower color, but within a population of plants both colors occur. It is striking how a desert species, so well adapted to minimize water loss, can put on such a showy—and water wasting—display of flowers. The spines are generally shorter than those on the grizzly bear cactus, and its pads have noticeably fewer clusters of spines. *(blackbrush scrub* and *Mojave desert scrub)*

If you wish to learn more about the canyon's plants, *River and Desert Plants of the Grand Canyon* (see page 164) is an excellent reference. Also, pick up a copy of *Checklist of Selected Plants of the Grand Canyon Area* at any of the Grand Canyon Natural History Association bookstores.

## ANIMALS

As with plants, the large elevation gradient from river to rim and the intricacies of the canyon landscape that create numerous microenvironments mean that many species of animals exist within the park. All species must be able to tolerate—or avoid—the extreme temperatures present in the Grand Canyon. Many species of birds migrate to warmer environments in winter and during the summer months are only active at dawn and dusk, hiding in brush thickets or riparian areas during the day. In summer, most reptiles, amphibians, and small mammals emerge only at dawn, dusk, or at night, spending hot summer days underground; they hibernate during the winter months. Some mammals *estivate* (a term describing "hibernation" during hot times of the year). The species described below are, mostly, those that are active during the day and quite widespread in their habitat choice, such that an astute—and lucky—hiker is likely to observe many of them.

### *Mammals*

**Bats:** Although 10 species of bats are identified as "common" in the Grand Canyon, a casual observer would have a difficult time determining which set of fluttering wings she observes. The western pipistrelle is the bat most commonly seen feeding on insects at dawn and dusk in the vicinity of the Bright Angel Campground. Nesting in small crevices and caves in the canyon walls, they emerge at dusk to feed.

**Cliff chipmunk:** Approximately 8 inches long including its tail, this is the only species of chipmunk, that inhabits the canyon and can be seen scurrying across rocky areas throughout the day. Unlike the larger ground squirrels, chipmunks have stripes on their faces. The stripes on the cliff chipmunk's back are less distinct that those of species found on the North Rim.

**Rock squirrel:** This ground squirrel, approximately 18 inches long including its tail, is a common resident both inside the canyon and along the rims. Its coat is a mottled gray-brown, becoming a reddish-brown toward its tail, and its trailing tail is moderately fluffy. Active during the day, these critters are terrible beggars—please resist the temptation to feed them; it is illegal and encourages this pesky behavior.

**Antelope ground squirrel:** A well-adapted desert species, antelope ground squirrels are active throughout the day—in the hottest parts of the canyon. Approximately 8 inches long including their tail, they are easily identified by their tail, which is about half the length of their back and usually bent back against their back displaying the mostly white underside. Two white stripes decorate their back.

**Coyote:** The coyote is a ubiquitous species in the Southwest, occurring from low-elevation desert into the alpine zone. Moreover, this member of the dog family with a grayish-beige coat is frequently seen walking solitarily across the landscape, as it is active throughout the day.

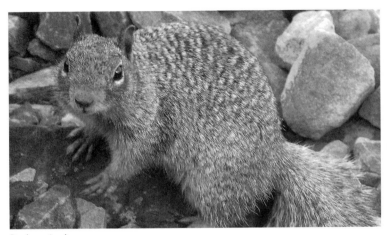

Rock squirrel

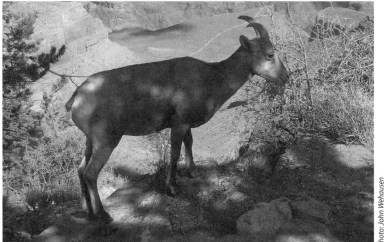

Photo: John Wehausen

Bighorn sheep

**Ringtail:** The ringtail, a relative of the raccoon, is a slender animal with a long black-and-white striped tail and a catlike face. It is common through much of the canyon below the rims, but especially in riparian corridors frequented by people, such as the campgrounds along the corridor trails. Until poles and food storage boxes were installed, these nocturnal creatures were nuisances, raiding food if hikers were inattentive or sleeping.

**Mule deer:** Mule deer inhabit the entire elevation range from rim to river. They tend to descend to river level only when there is insufficient food and water at higher elevations. At these times, they can be seen in any of the riparian corridors, feeding on leaves and any available patches of grass.

**Bighorn sheep:** Bighorn sheep occur throughout the canyon, scampering ably up cliffs that scare seasoned human scramblers. Despite being rather shy, bighorn sheep are regularly seen on both trails, especially near the summit of the Bright Angel Trail. They are even known to snack on the lovely green grass at the trailhead.

### Birds

Below are brief descriptions of 15 birds common to many of the Grand Canyon's habitats. This small sampling of the more than 300 species observed in the park is skewed to species active during the middle of the day and in particular to birds that will soar above you. Others are included because they are very common and quite easy to identify, especially important when you are steadily moving and not carrying binoculars.

**Turkey vulture:** Turkey vultures are a summer resident of the Grand Canyon that are frequently seen soaring on thermals. In flight, these large black birds are distinguishable from condors, hawks, and eagles by their V-shaped wing position and erratically tipping ("drunken") flight pattern.

**California condor:** Many mornings you can watch North America's largest bird, with a wingspan reaching 9 feet, warming their wings on pinnacles near the start of the Bright Angel Trail before soaring into the thermals. In addition to their much greater size, California

## REINTRODUCING THE CALIFORNIA CONDOR

Having a good shot at observing North America's largest land bird, the California condor, is a fantastic side benefit of a visit to the South Rim of the Grand Canyon. The wild populations had long been in decline due to pesticides, lead poisoning, and habitat destruction. They disappeared from Arizona by the 1930s and in 1987 the last wild birds were captured in California to bolster the captive breeding program. This program was very successful, and the first condors were reintroduced in California in 1992. Then in 1996 they were reintroduced to the Vermilion Cliffs, 30 miles north of the Grand Canyon.

Today there is a healthy population of 76 individuals on the Colorado Plateau, including a number who roost in the cliffs near the start of the Bright Angel Trail in summer. During the past few years chicks have been successfully reared in nests in the Grand Canyon. However, there does continue to be significant condor mortality. One culprit is the unintentional ingestion of metals, in the form of lead bullets (in carrion on which the birds feed) and coins (in particular those dropped below the rim of the Grand Canyon by tourists). Heed the signs posted along the rim and don't donate your coins to the canyon.

condors can be distinguished from turkey vultures by their flatter wings, white triangular patches beneath their wings, and lack of side-to-side tipping during flight. Their wingspan is approximately one and a half times that of the turkey vulture.

**Red-tailed hawk:** This easily identified hawk is very common throughout North America. Its distinct reddish tail is rapidly seen in a bird either perched on a tree or soaring. They hunt for small mammals in open areas; the Tonto Platform and the canyon rim are both ideal habitat for the red-tailed hawk.

**Golden eagle:** This large species also graces skies above the Grand Canyon. With a wingspan between 6 and 7 feet, the golden eagle is slightly larger than the turkey vulture. Although similar in shape to the much smaller hawks, it is much more darkly colored than commonly observed hawks: Its belly and inner wing feathers (coverts) are mostly dark brown, with a stripe of white on its inner tail feather and patches of white near its wing tips.

**American kestrel:** Falcons inhabiting the Grand Canyon include the American kestrel, the peregrine falcon, and the prairie falcon. All falcons are distinguishable from hawks by their pointed wing tips, and the American kestrel is the smallest of the falcons. Both the male and female American kestrels have a rufous-barred back, but the male's wings are gray and the female's rufous. These birds are often seen perched on trees or agaves as they search for insects and small mammals to dine upon.

**Peregrine falcon and prairie falcon:** Considerably larger than the kestrel, these skilled aerial hunters are capable of diving for a small mammal or bird from either a perch or while soaring high above the ground. The prairie falcon is dull beige with light-colored undersides, while the peregrine falcon displays very elegant markings: distinct black lines below the eye, a black-and-white-barred breast, and slate-colored back. Peregrine falcon populations have thrived in the Grand Canyon, where steep walls offer protected nesting sites. And the tall cliffs mean that visitors might see this species, the fastest of North America's birds, diving rapidly.

**Gambel's quail:** A year-round resident of the southwestern U.S., Gambel's quail is found throughout the Grand Canyon and is the only quail present in the park. Usually seen in small family groups, it is easily identified by its plume; a large forward curving plume adorns the males, while the females have a smaller upright one.

**White-throated swift:** A summer resident throughout the Grand Canyon, white-throated swifts are ubiquitous aerial acrobats that feed on airborne insects. They can be distinguished from swallows by their somewhat larger size; slightly bent, pointed wings; and long tail. This species is identified by white patches on its plumage, especially its white throat. Their ceaseless twittering is heard throughout the descent into the canyon.

**Black-chinned hummingbird:** This summer resident can be seen feeding on flowers alongside the trail; their favorites are deep tubular flowers from which they extract nectar with their long bills. Agave blooms are one likely location to see them. The males are elegant with a bright purple throat and a bold black chin. The backs of both male and females are iridescent green.

**Say's phoebe:** A species of flycatcher, the Say's phoebe is a year-round resident in all Grand Canyon habitats except the North Rim. Commonly found perched in open settings, the Say's phoebe is identified by its short, broad bill (a trait shared by all flycatchers), light grayish throat and pale, reddish-brown belly. Unlike many flycatchers, the top of its head is distinctly noncrested.

**Common raven:** The common raven is a well-known nuisance at Grand Canyon campgrounds, including those in the backcountry: They rapidly raid any unattended food. Since this jet-black species occurs anywhere, you will likely see many on your descent. It is larger than a crow and is distinguished from the latter by its bill; a raven's bill is much thicker and has a more distinctly tapered tip.

**Violet-green swallow:** A summer resident along riparian corridors, the violet-green swallow is especially common along the Colorado River corridor; it prefers to feed above water in open areas, eating aerial insects. On rare occasions, large numbers may be seen foraging along Bright Angel Creek by the campground. Their bright green and purple tails are not easily visible in flying individuals, but the white cheek patch and white above the eye distinguish it from other swallows.

**Rock wren:** A year-round resident common in most canyon environments, the rock wren is similar in size to the canyon wren (see opposite). Two distinguishing features of this mottled gray-brown species are the thin white stripe above its eye and the reddish patch at the base of its tail. Like all wrens, it has a thin, chisel-shaped bill. Its preferred habitat is jumbled rock.

**Canyon wren:** The canyon wren can be difficult to spot, but it gives away its ubiquitous presence in canyons with an unmistakable call: a series of descending minor notes that give it a mournful presence. If seen, it is easily identified by its reddish coloration and white throat. This year-round Grand Canyon resident has an especially long and slightly curved bill, ideal for probing crevices in cliff walls for insects.

### Reptiles

**Grand Canyon rattlesnake:** This subspecies of the western rattle-snake has evolved coloration to match the pinkish sand that forms from several of the rock strata. Like all rattlesnakes it is venomous, has a triangular head, and shakes a series of rattles on its tail to warn of its presence when threatened. Although this species is present in most habitats below the canyon rim, it avoids the main corridors, so you are unlikely to encounter it along the trails described here. Do not pick up a rattlesnake—or any other snake, since it's easy to misidentify them—most bites occur on the hands of people attempting to pick up a snake.

**Gopher snake:** A common snake found from approximately the Tonto Platform to the canyon rims, the gopher snake has indistinct beige and brown stripes along its back and a round head. Individuals of this harmless snake can reach 9 feet in length. When disturbed, it can mimic a rattlesnake, shaking its (rattle-less) tail.

**Collared lizard:** Its neck collar, two stripes of black with white in-between, easily identifies this species. About 8 inches long, including their tail, collared lizards often have beautiful coloration, with males displaying striking orange sides during breeding season. Their preferred habitat is dry slopes with some small rock cover.

**Chuckwalla:** These large dark lizards have enormous, flattened bellies—filled with plant matter, for they are vegetarians; including their tail, they are usually more than a foot long. Like all lizards, chuckwallas can tolerate the midday heat and can be found basking atop large boulders.

Pick up a copy of *Checklist of the Wildlife of the Grand Canyon* at any of the Grand Canyon Natural History Association bookstores for additional information.

# Grand Canyon Region Weather

The Grand Canyon is situated within the southern Colorado Plateau, a semiarid region with biseasonal rainfall peaks (winter and summer) and large daily and yearly shifts in temperature. These shape when hiking conditions are most comfortable—spring and fall—and indicate that hikers will experience an enormous range of temperatures on even a two-day hike to the river and back. A quick look at the climate data from the South Rim and Phantom Ranch (see below and pages 50–51) show daily swings of 20° to 35°F, yearly shifts of up to 50°F in average highs, and 20° to 30°F variation from canyon rim to river bottom. Desert areas experience large swings in temperature because of the low amount of moisture in the soil; water buffers temperature change because it requires a much greater input of heat for a given temperature change than something dry—and soil is a large moisture reservoir. The rainfall pattern reflects the two weather systems that influence the region: winter frontal storms originating in the Pacific Ocean and the summer monsoon, moisture derived from the Gulf of California (and beyond).

## TEMPERATURES AND PRECIPITATION AT THE SOUTH RIM

| | JAN | FEB | MARCH | APRIL | MAY |
|---|---|---|---|---|---|
| **Average High** (°F/°C) | 44 / 7 | 47 / 8 | 52 / 11 | 60 / 16 | 70 / 21 |
| **Average Low** (°F/°C) | 18 / -8 | 21 / -6 | 24 / -4 | 29 / -2 | 35 / 2 |
| **Record High** (°F/°C) | 71 / 22 | 69 / 21 | 74 / 23 | 82 / 28 | 92 / 33 |
| **Record Low** (°F/°C) | -17 / -27 | -20 / -29 | -1 / -18 | 8 / -13 | 17 / -8 |
| **Average Precipitation** (inches) | 1.78 | 1.61 | 2.02 | 1 | 0.59 |
| **Precipitation** (one-day maximum) | 1.16 | 1.41 | 1.44 | 1.4 | 0.65 |

**Note:** Figures are averages for 1976 to 2006.
Data is derived from www.wrcc.dri.edu/summary/climsmaz.html.

Overall, the climate data indicate that hikers need to choose different gear, hike during different hours of the day, and simply have different expectations based on the month of their visit—and the weather forecast. The latter is important, for averages are simply averages, and the temperatures on any given day can range far from the norm. For instance, I have twice had the "privilege" of arriving on the South Rim of the Grand Canyon for a cold, snowy Memorial Day and found that hiking in the Inner Gorge was still tolerably cool midmorning.

A quick march through the seasons should help you plan:

**Winter:** By late fall, large, moist low-pressure systems are reaching the western U.S., depositing much moisture along the coast and continuing inland. These extensive systems can deposit widespread snow to the rims of the Grand Canyon and rain along the Colorado River. The trajectory of the storms—and therefore whether they impact the Grand Canyon—is dictated by the position of the jet stream, and the amount of moisture they contain when they

| JUNE | JULY | AUG | SEPT | OCT | NOV | DEC |
|------|------|-----|------|-----|-----|-----|
| 81 / 27 | 85 / 29 | 82 / 28 | 76 / 24 | 64 / 18 | 52 / 11 | 45 / 7 |
| 43 / 6 | 50 / 10 | 49 / 9 | 43 / 6 | 33 / 1 | 24 / -4 | 18 / -8 |
| 95 / 35 | 101 / 38 | 96 / 36 | 93 / 34 | 83 / 28 | 72 / 22 | 65 / 18 |
| 25 / -4 | 35 / 2 | 36 / 2 | 24 / -4 | 8 / -13 | -6 / -21 | -20 / -29 |
| 0.4 | 1.92 | 2.18 | 1.52 | 1.28 | 1.36 | 1.17 |
| 1.1 | 3.14 | 3.28 | 2.56 | 2.08 | 1.95 | 1.71 |

## TEMPERATURES AND PRECIPITATION
## IN THE INNER GORGE AT PHANTOM RANCH

| | JAN | FEB | MARCH | APRIL | MAY |
|---|---|---|---|---|---|
| Average High (°F/°C) | 57 / 14 | 64 / 18 | 72 / 22 | 82 / 28 | 92 / 33 |
| Average Low (°F/°C) | 37 / 3 | 42 / 6 | 47 / 8 | 54 / 12 | 63 / 17 |
| Record High (°F/°C) | 81 / 27 | 83 / 28 | 93 / 34 | 106 / 41 | 111 / 44 |
| Record Low (°F/°C) | -9 / -23 | 21 / -6 | 25 / -4 | 28 / -2 | 32 / 0 |
| Average Precipitation (inches) | 3.17 | 3.22 | 2.65 | 1.73 | 1.17 |
| Precipitation (one-day maximum) | 1.3 | 1.3 | 1 | 0.87 | 0.68 |

**Note:** Figures are averages for 1966 to 2006.
Data is derived from www.wrcc.dri.edu/summary/climsmaz.html.

reach the Colorado Plateau determines the severity of the storm. Temperatures are chilly throughout winter, especially since steep walls mean the sun penetrates much of the inner canyon for only a few hours each day.

**Spring:** During March and April nighttime lows are still below freezing on the South Rim, but daytime temperatures are pleasant and sometimes hot throughout the canyon. By April, the Pacific storms have mostly abated and much less precipitation falls in the region. May brings much hotter temperatures, and during warm periods the Inner Gorge is already much too hot for midday hiking.

**Summer:** Summer is the season of intense heat in the Grand Canyon, especially in the Inner Gorge. Not only do midday temperatures far exceed 100°F, but also the dark rock absorbs and reradiates the heat. Nighttime temperatures in the Inner Gorge remain high as the dark rock continues to radiate heat all night. During these months, plan to walk at the lowest elevations only at dawn

| JUNE | JULY | AUG | SEPT | OCT | NOV | DEC |
|------|------|------|------|------|------|------|
| 103 / 39 | 106 / 41 | 103 / 39 | 96 / 36 | 83 / 28 | 68 / 20 | 57 / 14 |
| 72 / 22 | 77 / 25 | 74 / 23 | 68 / 20 | 58 / 14 | 46 / 8 | 38 / 3 |
| 119 / 48 | 120 / 49 | 120 / 49 | 110 / 43 | 102 / 39 | 87 / 31 | 77 / 25 |
| 50 / 10 | 60 / 16 | 59 / 15 | 48 / 9 | 40 / 4 | 19 / -7 | 12 / -11 |
| 0.86 | 1.93 | 2.85 | 1.99 | 1.38 | 1.48 | 2.83 |
| 0.51 | 1.85 | 1.66 | 2.65 | 1.55 | 1.84 | 1.55 |

and dusk, resting in the shade or escaping to higher elevations by a few hours after sunrise.

By early July the subtropical North American Monsoon (see page 52) is delivering moisture across northern Mexico and into the southwestern U.S., including thunderstorms in the Grand Canyon region. In the Grand Canyon, the greatest danger associated with these thunderstorms is flash flooding, as water drains rapidly through the porous soils and over rock, funneling into small drainages (see page 66). The extent of cloud cover and rainfall can be very patchy, with several inches of moisture falling in one drainage and none a few miles away. Moreover, the section of a drainage where you are hiking might have received no rainfall, but rain may have fallen in upstream areas; be attentive to conditions—and avoid washes—anytime you suspect rainfall in the region. Lightning is mostly a concern only if you are on the canyon rim or a large open expanse, but it is also wise to avoid ridge trails during intense thunderstorm activity (see page 67).

## THE NORTH AMERICAN MONSOON

The North American Monsoon begins to develop in late spring, as intense heating over the deserts of northern Mexico and the southwestern U.S. create a surface low-pressure area and upper atmosphere high-pressure region. Wind directions in the upper atmosphere shift from a westerly to a southeasterly or easterly direction. As a result, low-level moisture is drawn in from the Gulf of California and the eastern Pacific, to the south, and high-level moisture flows from the Gulf of Mexico, to the southeast, encircling the high pressure in a clockwise direction.

Initially, storms produce little rainfall, as the moisture reevaporates before reaching the ground, but by early July the lower levels of the atmosphere are sufficiently moist that ever more rainfall reaches the surface.

The amount of moisture in the region, and therefore thunderstorm activity, varies during the monsoon. If the high-pressure ridge moves south or east, less moisture is drawn over Arizona and thunderstorm activity diminishes. In contrast, especially large amounts of moisture can enter the region when remnants of tropical storms are carried north. The North American Monsoon is much stronger in southern Arizona than on the Colorado Plateau.

For more information, see the excellent website maintained by the Tucson office of the National Weather Service: www.wrh.noaa.gov/twc/monsoon/monsoon_info.php.

**Fall:** By mid-September, cold fronts are again approaching the Pacific coast, and the wind direction over the Grand Canyon region reverts to a westerly or northwesterly flow. With this shift, the monsoon ends, and drier conditions exist over the Grand Canyon. Temperatures are milder, but still pleasant and warm, making late September and October popular months to backpack in the Grand Canyon. During October and November, keep your eye on the forecast, so the first winter storm does not take you by surprise.

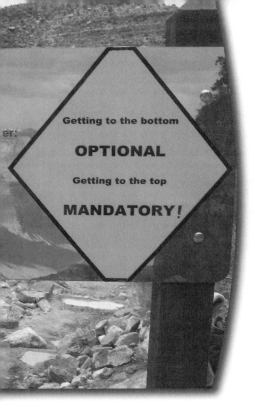

Getting to the bottom

**OPTIONAL**

Getting to the top

**MANDATORY!**

# 2
# Precautions and Considerations

**A**ny wilderness activity exposes you to the risk of injury, or even death, because you are pushing yourself physically and exposing yourself to potentially extreme climate and weather conditions. Moreover, there are no readily available medical facilities. Hikers in the Grand Canyon are especially likely to have medical problems, mostly from a combination of descending first and the hot conditions during much of the year. As a result, the rangers in the Grand Canyon are, with good reason, exceptionally vehement in their admonition not to descend past Plateau Point (on the Bright Angel Trail) or Skeleton Point (on the South Kaibab Trail) while dayhiking, even in cool weather.

There have been approximately 100 recorded accidental deaths of people hiking below the rim on the Grand Canyon's trails—and many more on the rim, on the river, on aerial tours, and while hiking off-trail. Of those, around 60 have occurred on the South Kaibab and Bright Angel trails. This number is relatively low in comparison to the enormous number of visitors—and that is

*Above:* One of the ubiquitous park service reminders that you must ascend whatever you descend

## GETTING TO THE BOTTOM, OPTIONAL. GETTING TO THE TOP, MANDATORY!

As you read the precautions and considerations, keep in mind the mantra posted throughout the park: "Getting to the bottom, optional. Getting to the top, mandatory!" Unlike hiking in a mountain range, when entering a canyon you begin your excursion by heading down. Two of the important implications are: (1) Temperatures increase rapidly as you go down, because you are descending in elevation as the day heats up. Consequently, you end up at the lowest, hottest part of your hike at midday. (2) You are unlikely to get tired on the way down and do not realize you have overextended yourself until you are at the bottom.

thanks to the vigilance and heroic efforts of park rangers and fellow hikers. Consider that between 2000 and 2009 there were 3,284 rescues on the Bright Angel and South Kaibab trails, suggesting that the number of deaths caused by environmental conditions could be much, much higher and that many hikers have put themselves in unacceptable positions because they did not understand weather conditions and their own capabilities.

Large numbers of people visit the South Rim during the heat of summer. Some of them ignore the warnings and assume that they are fitter and more heat tolerant than those who have been rescued. You can avoid becoming part of these statistics by considering the dangers you face and keeping your body cool, well hydrated, and well fed. And, take solace realizing that more people have died while on aerial sightseeing tours than through other hazards in the Grand Canyon, including rafting accidents and falls from the canyon rim.

## Hyponatremia

Hyponatremia, or water intoxication, caused by too low a level of sodium in the blood, is one of the health risks faced by Grand Canyon hikers. The conditions experienced while hiking the Grand Canyon are exactly those that are most associated with hyponatremia: hot weather and an exercise "event" that lasts more than four hours. In particular, hikers will suffer from "exercise-associated hyponatremia," indicating that exercise, not an underlying physiological disorder, is causing the sodium ion depletion.

While the following section focuses on hyponatremia, insufficient levels of many other ions can also occur. In particular, potassium (hypokalemia), chlorine (hypochloremia), magnesium (hypomagnesemia), and calcium (hypocalcemia) can all become depleted. The many different essential ions are collectively termed electrolytes. Each type of ion plays an important role in the body's physiology. For instance, sodium ions are important for the transmission of electrical signals between nerve cells and for heart activity. Total electrolyte depletion is also a problem because water is drawn from the blood stream into surrounding tissues, potentially causing severe problems like cerebral edema, the swelling of the brain.

## CAUSES

Hyponatremia is usually caused simply by drinking too much water: Our kidneys can process at most a little more than a quart (one liter) per hour. If we consume water in excess of total water loss (the sum of maximal kidney function plus the water we sweat out and lose through breathing, see page 61 for more information), our body will become overhydrated.

Loss of sodium ions through sweat is a second mechanism that leads to lower sodium ion concentrations: Two grams of sodium can be lost with each liter of water evaporated as sweat. While sweating exacerbates the effects of overhydration, it has not been documented as being the actual cause of hyponatremia: There is no difference in sodium ion loss between athletes who develop hyponatremia and those who do not. (However, note that as a Grand Canyon hiker, you are out in the hot sun sweating for even more hours than the marathon runners on whom these statistics are gathered.)

## SYMPTOMS

Officially, hyponatremia is defined as a decrease in sodium ion concentration to less than 135 millimoles of ions per liter of blood. However sodium ion levels differ among people, and in general a decrease of 7 to 10 percent in sodium ions concentration leads to hyponatremia symptoms. The first symptoms include bloating, puffiness, nausea, vomiting, and headache. If the condition worsens, brain swelling, altered mental state, respiratory distress, and eventually a coma and death can result. Note that women and people with a low body weight are more susceptible to hyponatremia.

## PREVENTION

It is important not to drink excessive amounts of water—for most people no more than three-quarters of a quart (0.7 liter) per hour—and to eat salty snacks. While most people will continue drinking fluids—as long as they don't run out—many hikers consume far too little food during their excursion into the Grand Canyon and eat less and less if they begin to feel sick from the heat. Moreover, many people assume that they can substitute electrolyte drinks for food—a misconception, since many sports drinks have low sodium concentrations. It is important that you carry a variety of snacks,

### MAINTAINING HOMEOSTASIS

The human body is a carefully regulated machine, maintaining a near-constant temperature, water content, blood sugar level, and stable concentration of sodium ions, potassium ions, and many other ions. The body uses physiological processes, both chemical and physical in nature, to maintain a stable internal environment, a concept known as homeostasis. The beauty of the system is that our body, within certain boundaries, can maintain homeostasis even though the external temperature varies and we do not eat and drink continuously or in the *exact* proportions our body requires.

This careful balancing act can, however, be disrupted. Yes, the body uses physiological processes to *fine-tune* temperature, water content, blood sugar, and ion levels. However, these physiological processes require that we provide approximately the correct amount of heat input (or loss), water, and food. If we do not provide appropriate inputs, the body has some simple ways of telling us it is having trouble maintaining homeostasis: headaches, nausea, muscle cramps, and eventually an altered mental state. Since these same symptoms are the result of lots of different "problems," it can be difficult to self-diagnose a specific cause. If you develop one while pushing yourself through exercise, sit down, eat food, drink water, and rest so that your body can reestablish its balance.

so that something looks appetizing no matter how tired you are (see page 92 for suggestions). Of course if you develop a headache, nausea, or muscle cramps, you might also be dehydrated and vulnerable to heat exhaustion and heatstroke—keep reading!

# Dehydration

Dehydration occurs when your body has less water and other fluids than it should, when water intake is less than combined water loss due to sweating, breathing, and urination. Symptoms include a dry, sticky mouth, thirst, a headache, fatigue, and muscle weakness. Mild dehydration can readily be treated by increasing fluid consumption, including drinking fluids containing electrolytes. Dehydration is especially a concern, because untreated dehydration leads to heat illnesses, including heat exhaustion and heatstroke. If you suspect a group member is dehydrated, take a break in the shade and consume lots of fluids and a large snack.

# Heat Illnesses

Heat exhaustion and heatstroke are two distinct heat-related emergencies. Heat exhaustion is a more easily treatable problem caused by dehydration and electrolyte depletion and leading to slight increases in body temperature. If heat exhaustion is not treated, the body temperature rises to the point that it can no longer regulate itself, a life-threatening emergency known as heatstroke.

These illnesses occur due to exercise on a hot day (which heats the body up) in combination with insufficient intake of fluids and electrolytes (which restricts the body's main cooling mechanism, sweating). To avoid heat illness, consume sufficient liquid and food, thereby providing the water needed to sweat. Also, you can minimize your susceptibility to heat illnesses by acclimatizing yourself to exercising in a hot environment over a period of two to three weeks. Starting with just 15 to 20 minutes of exercise per day, work your way up to at least an hour per day. Heat acclimatization includes physiological changes such as increased sweat production, improving your ability to cool yourself (see page 83 for additional information).

## HEAT PRODUCTION AND LOSS

Humans, like all mammals, are warm-blooded or homoeothermic, meaning we maintain a constant body temperature of approximately 98.6°F. Our bodies perform best at this temperature and will shut down if our internal temperature increases above 104°F or decreases below 90°F (for more about hypothermia, see page 62). The balance between metabolic heat production, environmental heat gain, and various mechanisms of heat loss determines whether our body temperature remains around 98.6°F.

We produce our own heat primarily by metabolizing food; our combustion engines are much more efficient than a car, but 60 percent of our food still gets converted into heat, not usable energy. You burn about 8 calories per minute while hiking uphill carrying a daypack and 10 calories per minute while hiking with an overnight pack. A backpacker therefore burns 600 calories per hour, creating 360 calories of heat. (The number of calories burned varies enormously by person. These are values for a fit 150-pound person.)

As homeotherms, we then need to shed that heat to maintain a constant body temperature. Perspiring—and having that sweat evaporate—is the most effective way to lose heat, especially in dry climates. Your body heat causes the sweat to evaporate, in the process leaving you cooler. (In a humid climate sweating is less effective, because the air is already mostly saturated with water molecules and the water on your skin evaporates at a slower rate.) For each quart (liter) of sweat that evaporates the body uses 580

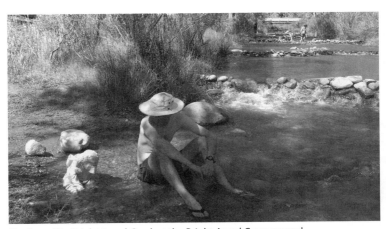

Cooling off in Bright Angel Creek at the Bright Angel Campground heat calories. Therefore if you are creating 360 calories of heat per hour, losing approximately 0.6 quart (0.6 liter) of sweat per hour will offset this heat increase. We can also shed heat by increasing blood flow to peripheral regions (i.e., fingers and toes) or decrease peripheral blood flow to minimize heat loss. Unless our body runs out of water or heats up *too quickly*, it can effectively adjust sweat production and blood flow to shed the necessary amount of heat.

When extra water is available, we can artificially augment our "sweat" by wetting our clothes; water evaporating from our clothes cools the body nearly as effectively as the evaporation of sweat and doesn't use up our body's water or salts. Either creek or tap water can be used for this purpose.

We can also gain heat from or lose heat to the environment through three other physical processes: radiation, convection, and conduction.

**Radiation** is energy that is emitted from an object in the form of electromagnetic waves, such as the heat we receive from the sun. All substances radiate heat, including people, trees, and the earth, and the amount of heat they radiate is a function of their temperature. If the temperature of substances around us is lower than our body temperature, we experience a net heat loss. In contrast, on a sunny summer day, incoming radiation can increase our heat input by 300 calories per hour, nearly the amount of heat produced by hiking uphill—additional heat we need to lose through sweating.

**Convection** is the transfer of heat away from (or to) a body, because the molecules move: for instance, when air molecules near our skin are heated and then moved away by the wind, new (cooler) air molecules are brought near our skin. This process is more effective in people with a high surface area to volume ratio (i.e., skinny people) because they have more surface area to disperse it. Convective heat loss is higher on windy days. Fanning is a method of artificially increasing convective heat loss. Lightweight, loose-fitting clothes promote convective heat loss by increasing airflow. And light-colored clothes keep you cooler in the first place (see more about light-colored clothing on page 96). And lying down in a cold creek, such as Garden or Bright Angel creeks, is an excellent way to experience convective heat loss.

**Conduction** is the transfer of heat from one molecule to the next, such as heat transferred from (or to) our skin surface to (or from) a solid or liquid. The only conductive heat transfer hikers experience is through their feet—if your shoe soles are too thin, your feet might get hot or cold—and hardly affects heat balance.

## HEAT EXHAUSTION

Heat exhaustion is generally caused either by dehydration or by electrolyte depletion, both of which occur through exercise. If we are dehydrated or our electrolytes are depleted, the body's ability to sweat will be compromised, decreasing its ability to regulate temperature. Symptoms include a rapid and weak pulse, fatigue, increased sweating, and eventually disorientation and fainting. A person displaying these symptoms should rest (in the shade if possible), drink water, and eat salty foods.

### HOW THE BODY USES WATER

You have probably heard various recommendations of how much water to consume, both while resting and exercising. A long-standing suggestion is that a fairly sedentary adult needs to drink two quarts (two liters) of liquids a day, in addition to the two cups (half liter) of water obtained from food. In addition, it is widely reported that you should drink one quart per hour—or as much as you can tolerate—while exercising. Ignoring the danger of hyponatremia for a moment, consider why (and if) this much water is required and how it is used by and then exits your body.

For starters, a human is 60 to 70 percent water, with leaner individuals having a higher percentage. Water fills our cells and the tissues that surround our cells. Electrolytes and various biological molecules are dissolved or suspended in water. The body requires a specific concentration of each molecule, and when it becomes dehydrated the concentration changes, leading to myriad physiological problems. A decrease in water content of even a few percentage points leads to dehydration.

Although our total water content remains fairly constant, the body continuously processes water. An average, healthy, but sedentary individual loses about 2.5 quarts (2.5 liters) of water each day: 6 cups (0.75 liter) through urination, 2 cups (0.5 liter) through sweating, a little more than

## HEATSTROKE

With continued exercise under hot conditions and insufficient water intake, heat exhaustion can progress to heatstroke. A very high body temperature (104°F or above) and changed neurological conditions are signs of heatstroke. Such a high body temperature causes the body to lose its ability to control body temperature and sweat, thereby making it even more vulnerable to environmental conditions. In other words, the body's negative feedback mechanism to regulate body temperature by sweating fails, and is replaced by a dangerous response: producing less sweat and therefore having less control of body temperature, when you are already too hot and sweating too little. It can develop quickly and requires immediate attention.

1 cup by exhaling, and 0.5 cup with your feces. In addition the body requires a small amount of water to metabolize the food we eat. Foods with more complex molecular structures and high protein foods, such as meat, require more water to digest, than those with simpler molecular structures, such as bread, but this effect is small compared to the body's other water requirements.

While exercising, especially in a hot, dry environment, water loss through sweating and breathing increase enormously. Moderate to hard exercise, such as hiking up a steep trail at a quick pace, can increase water loss through sweating and breathing to a quart (or a liter) per hour. (We lose water while breathing, for the air we breathe out is moister than what we breathe in, and with exercise this process can result in 0.3 quart (0.3 liter) of water loss per hour.) If our water intake is inadequate during exercise, the water content in our bloodstream and our tissues decreases, leading to dehydration. It is therefore tempting to consume ever more water if we exercise harder, especially in hot, dry conditions. However, the kidneys can process only a quart (a liter) per hour—overwhelming the kidneys or diluting ions and sugars in the blood can lead to overhydration or hyponatremia. Instead it is essential to reduce the intensity of exercise and take breaks.

Although heatstroke is most commonly caused by exercising in hot environments, dehydration, cardiovascular disease, and alcohol use also contribute to heatstroke. People taking certain medications, especially medications for psychological conditions, are at increased risk for heatstroke. Also, people who have recently had a heat illness are more vulnerable to another episode. Children are at especially high risk of heatstroke, since the ability to sweat does not develop fully until puberty. (Many fatalities in the Grand Canyon are caused by heart failure or heart attacks. In many cases the victim likely had a heart condition that was exacerbated by dehydration and exertion on a hot day, triggering a heart attack.)

In addition to an elevated body temperature, symptoms of heatstroke include hot and dry skin, rapid heartbeat and breathing, cessation of sweating, nausea, a headache, irritability (or simply a change in personality), and fainting (especially in older adults).

If you suspect that a party member has heatstroke, have her rest in the shade, drink cold water, cover her with moistened clothing, and fan her with moistened clothing. Remember that untreated water can be used to wet clothing—don't deplete your precious water supplies unnecessarily. If shade is unavailable, try to create some by spanning a tarp, tent rainfly, or clothing atop available vegetation.

## Hypothermia

Hypothermia is a potentially lethal condition that results from an abnormally low body temperature. Usually presumed to occur at cold temperatures, it can happen at an air temperature as high as 70°F, especially if the person is wet from rain or sweat and/or the conditions are windy. Although it may be difficult to accept that you could be too cold when visiting the Grand Canyon, it's a very real concern during the cooler months of the year, especially if it is raining or snowing. Even the Inner Gorge is mostly below 70°F from November to February, while the average high temperature on the South Rim rises above 70°F only from June to September and nighttime temperatures drop below freezing for more than half the year (see section on weather, page 48).

Hypothermia can occur with little warning and rapidly leads to a loss of mental function, which is why you must be aware of the early symptoms. Hypothermia sets in when your core body temperature drops below 95°F, only a 3.6-degree decrease from normal. The first symptom is shivering—the body's attempt to rewarm itself. Signs of confusion and difficulty speaking may occur when the core temperature drops below 94°F. In the advanced stages of hypothermia, shivering stops, the body's core temperature drops below 90°F, and a person may no longer feel cold. He or she will become incoherent, with severely limited judgment. Death can result if your body temperature drops below 80°F.

Mild hypothermia can be treated in the field, while severe hypothermia must to be treated in a medical facility so the patient can be rewarmed properly. Since poor heart function and sudden cardiac death is possible if a severely hypothermic patient is not handled carefully, it's imperative to catch and reverse mild hypothermia before it worsens.

If an injury (or poor planning) forces you to spend a night out, your clothes get wet in a storm, or you are underdressed on a cold, windy day, you are at severe risk of hypothermia.

Minimize your chances of becoming hypothermic by following these suggestions:

- Wear a hat. Much heat loss occurs through the head.
- If you end up with wet clothes, change into dry clothes immediately.
- If you are waiting for group members and start getting cold, put on extra clothes, move out of the wind, and pace back and forth, swinging your arms and legs vigorously to enhance circulation.

If you suspect someone in your group is hypothermic:

- Get him into a location sheltered from the wind.
- Make sure he is wearing warm, dry clothes.
- If the patient is conscious and can swallow, feed him warm, sweet liquids or easily digested foods.
- Put the hypothermic person in a pre-warmed sleeping bag, with warm water bottles placed inside.
- Monitor the patient's pulse, breathing, and body temperature (if possible). Plan to evacuate if the patient does not improve. If the condition is severe, get help immediately. Also remember that a severely hypothermic patient may appear to lack a pulse, but that does not mean the person is deceased.

# Falling

The two best ways to avoid falling and injuring yourself on the long descent are to walk slowly and to use trekking poles. Walking slowly puts less force on your knee with each step, and using trekking poles takes some weight off your knees and lessens your chances of falling. And a bizarre suggestion: Turning around to walk down those occasional really tall steps backward, especially if you're wearing a heavy pack, will significantly reduce the pressure on your knees by employing the stronger muscles of your upper legs. While I can't tell you how much this approach reduces strain on your knees, it helps me tremendously, and I have converted many friends. Also, if you have recurrent knee problems, wear a knee brace. Ensuring your hiking shoes or boots have good tread (see page 93) will also reduce your chances of falling and injuring yourself.

After an injury anti-inflammatory drugs (such as ibuprofen or naproxen) may alleviate the pain. You may choose to wrap your knee or ankle with the elastic bandage in your first-aid kit, but don't wrap it too tightly—restricting blood flow can exacerbate the injury. In fact, taping your ankle with sports tape is better than using an elastic bandage, as the elastic bandage will provide less stability and support and most people wrap them too tightly. Assess how badly you have injured yourself before deciding whether to continue your downward journey, retreat upward, or seek medical assistance and an evacuation.

While most falls on the Bright Angel and South Kaibab trails are not life-endangering injuries, the steep landscape makes fatal falls a possibility. Eight people have died from falls from (and near) the Bright Angel and South Kaibab trails. Most were people wandering off-trail to take photos or clown around, but some falls are unexplained. Heat exhaustion, heatstroke, or hyponatremia can all lead to altered consciousness, which could in turn lead to poor footing choices—or a choice to leave the trail and take a shortcut.

# Blisters

Even with broken-in, comfortable shoes, it is easy to get blisters when descending into and ascending from the bottom of the Grand Canyon. On your descent you are most likely to develop blisters on your toes and under the balls of your feet; the persistent downward motion tends to thrust your feet against the front of your shoes. In contrast, during the ascent, your heels will likely slip more in your boots, causing blisters to form on them. There are many tricks to minimize the severity of blisters and to tackle hot spots as soon as they begin to form. For instance:

- Wear the same shoes you wore on your training hikes (see the section on footwear, page 93).
- Wear well-padded, non-cotton, dry socks. If you are especially prone to sweaty feet, bring an extra pair of socks to switch into halfway up the climb. Some people wear two pairs of socks: a thin liner sock, usually made of polypropylene, and a thicker outer sock, made of wool or a wool-synthetic blend.
- Cover potential hot spots with tape (sports tape or other) or moleskin (see the first-aid kit section on page 98), either before you start or as soon as you sense a hot spot forming. Use pieces of tape long enough so that they don't fall off your heel.

The book *Lightweight Backpacking and Camping* by Ryan Jordan has many suggestions for reducing the possibility of injuries, especially blisters. Preventive measures include treating your feet with rubbing alcohol for the week before a long hike to toughen your foot and applying Tuf-Skin to your feet before your walk.

If a blister should develop, treat it promptly. Air your foot to dry the skin before applying a bandage. Some people are content covering small blisters with a piece of sports tape, but it is often better to apply blister bandages or a piece of moleskin, followed by sports tape. An old trick is to cut a piece of moleskin into a doughnut shape, such that a raised ring of moleskin surrounds the blister. However, many people now use blister bandages, which are quick to apply and will stay put for the remainder of your hike. Large blisters are best drained with a sterile pin before patching. Blisters on toes can be very difficult to treat, as taping one toe often causes a blister on the neighboring toe when the tape (or other blister treatment) rubs. Another option is to tape a toe blister with thin tape to minimize rubbing and to proactively tape the neighboring toe.

## Flash Floods

Flash floods are common in deserts, environments where locally concentrated, drenching thunderstorms are possible and only a thin layer of soil overlies the bedrock. Since the water cannot drain into the soil, it instead flows rapidly into small gullies and then coalesces into larger creek beds, which can flood without warning. Narrow canyons with steep walls are especially dangerous, because escape is impossible, but any desert wash is susceptible to flooding. Moreover, a flash flood is not simply a gush of water, but instead (usually) a slurry of mud, rocks, branches, and anything else that was lying in the wash—you are as likely to be killed by blunt force injuries as drowning.

Although flash floods are possible at any time, they are most likely during the summer monsoon. The highest single-day rainfall totals for the Grand Canyon (excluding rare winter storms on the North Rim) are during July through September: On August 29, 1951, 4.25 inches of rain fell at the Bright Angel Ranger Station on the North Rim, and on August 13, 2001, 3.28 inches of rain fell on the South Rim of the Grand Canyon. A warm winter storm can also cause flooding, for the pounding rain will melt snow, further increasing runoff.

### ACCIDENTS IN THE GRAND CANYON

If you are intrigued by the stories of how people have died from—or nearly succumbed to—various dangers in the Grand Canyon, pick up a copy of *Over the Edge: Death in the Grand Canyon* by Michael Ghiglieri and Thomas Myers. This encyclopedic account of fatal accidents (and intentional deaths) is full of outstanding descriptions of the environmental and medical conditions that led to the emergencies. It is both sobering and informative, driving home the power of nature and how important it is to know what not to do and when to be most cautious. They emphasize that a disproportionate number of victims are male and younger than age 30, implying that inappropriate risk-taking contributes to more accidents than unexpected conditions. The authors also include details of near-fatal mishaps, demonstrating the role luck can play.

Summer thunderstorms are especially dangerous, because you are often unaware of the danger: Because thunderstorms are patchy, nearby locations can receive vastly different amounts of rain. You may remain dry, while an upstream area rapidly receives multiple inches of rainfall. It is therefore necessary to be aware of the forecast for the entire region and if thunderstorms are forecast, assume water is falling somewhere, be especially vigilant, and don't take risks. Take your breaks away from the water's edge, and move quickly if you hear an odd thundering noise, akin to an approaching train.

The catchments draining the north side of the Grand Canyon, are often large, and you might not even see the clouds emptying themselves onto the upstream landscape, including portions of the Kaibab Plateau. Bright Angel Creek, flowing past the Bright Angel Campground, is one such location, where unknowing parties have been warned of an impending flood just in time. People exploring upstream from the campground, including Ribbon Falls along the North Kaibab Trail and in Phantom Canyon have been caught and killed by floods. The south side catchments are smaller, since water falling on the South Rim flows away from the canyon, but do not be complacent. A flash flood killed a father and son in 1963 on the Bright Angel Trail, a little upstream of Indian Garden. Since the South Kaibab Trail predominantly follows a ridge and broad slopes not gullies, it is not prone to flash floods.

# Lightning

Despite frequent summer thunderstorms, there have been very few fatalities in the Grand Canyon caused by lightning strikes. The handful of victims, including those who were injured and survived, were located in exposed places: at vista points on the canyon rim or on hiking trails that followed ridges, such as the South Kaibab Trail. Nonetheless, it is important to know how to protect yourself against lightning. If you are sightseeing from the canyon rim when a storm approaches, immediately seek shelter away from the canyon rim—and its metal barriers—in a building or a car. If there is not a shelter nearby, follow the precautions described below. If you are hiking on an exposed ridge, descend a short distance from the ridgeline (if possible) to wait until the storm passes, and follow the advice below:

- Stay out of shallow caves and away from overhangs.

- Get in the lightning position, both to reduce the likelihood of a direct strike and to reduce the seriousness of injury you are likely to sustain. The National Outdoor Leadership School recommends squatting or sitting as low as possible and wrapping your arms around your legs. This position minimizes your body's surface area, reducing the chances for a ground current to flow through you. Close your eyes, and keep your feet together to prevent the current from flowing in one foot and out the other.
- Squat on an insulated pad or a pile of clothes.

Should a member of your party be struck by lightning and stop breathing, immediately begin CPR. CPR is more likely to be successful following a lightning strike than many other injuries, as the electrical shock can stop a person's heart from beating without actually causing much internal damage. Indeed, 80 percent of strikes are not fatal. But be prepared to continue CPR or rescue breathing until medical professionals arrive.

## Scorpions

Bark scorpions (*Centruroides sculpturatus*) live under the bark of cottonwood trees, including those in Bright Angel Campground, as well as under rocks and in woodpiles. As long as three inches but commonly much shorter, these light brown scorpions are abundant in riparian areas and are unfortunately the most poisonous of North America's scorpions. They deliver a very painful sting comprised of a medley of neurotoxins causing severe pain for 24 to 72 hours. Adults are unlikely to be endangered by the bite, but it can be fatal for babies and young children. Fortunately, no Grand Canyon visitor has ever been killed by their sting, although during summer one in 200 visitors is stung. A ranger I met at the Bright Angel Campground considered it a stamp of experience that he had been bitten many times. (In Mexico, children occasionally die from scorpion stings, but the last fatality in Arizona was in 1964.)

To reduce the chance of spending a day of your vacation in agony, consider the following. You are most likely to encounter scorpions during the hot midsummer months, when they emerge at night to wander around and possibly join you in your sleeping liner or hide in your shoes or clothes. Many seasoned Grand Canyon hikers opt to take a mesh tent or sleep atop picnic tables during these months to avoid a nasty surprise. Second, shake out your belongings in the morning. Phantom Ranch guests are more likely to be bitten because the scorpions can squeeze into the cabins more easily than a zipped tent.

If you are bitten, taking an over-the-counter pain medication, such as aspirin, ibuprofen, naproxen, or acetaminophen will reduce the pain somewhat.

# Waterborne Pests

It is quite feasible to complete a walk on the Bright Angel and South Kaibab trails without ever needing to purify water: Along the Bright Angel Trail, piped water is available at 1.5-Mile Resthouse, 3-Mile Resthouse, and Indian Garden. Along the South Kaibab Trail, neither piped nor free-flowing water is available. And there are spigots at the Bright Angel Campground. In winter, spigots at the 1.5-Mile Resthouse and 3-Mile Resthouse are turned off, necessitating that you carry more water.

However, should you need to obtain water from another source, filter and then purify—or boil—it before consuming it. The protozoa *Giardia* and *Cryptosporidium* and the bacteria *E. coli* are all present in the Colorado River. At times, bacteria and protozoa contaminate many of the Grand Canyon's side tributaries, including Pipe, Garden, and Bright Angel creeks, and it is recommended that you filter all water sources, including those that are running clear.

Silt particles should be removed from water before chemical purification—an extra purification step necessary in desert environments, since silt can interfere with some purification processes and clog filters. Options include letting water settle undisturbed for many hours (i.e., overnight), pouring it through a coffee filter, or adding a clearing agent (i.e., aluminum sulfate, or alum) that causes the silt to settle quickly.

The second step is to kill or remove the microbes present. Possible methods include:

- **Chemical purification (e.g., iodine or chlorine):** This is the easiest method of treating water—simply add drops or a tablet—but you have to wait at least 20 minutes to drink your water, and it will be left with a distinct chemical flavor. In

## HIGH- AND LOW-FLOW WATERWAYS

An interesting National Park Service guideline indicates the difference in managing water quality along the Colorado River corridor versus the side creeks. They request that along the Colorado River you pee *in* the river *not* on the sand to prevent algal growth on the beaches. Your urine is instantly diluted in the Colorado River and does not affect its quality. In contrast, the low water flow in the side creeks makes it important to urinate away from these water sources.

addition, chemical purification kills *Cryptosporidium* only after many hours.

- **Water filter:** Water filters should remove all bacteria and protozoa, but the pores are too large to remove viruses, thankfully a minimal concern in this environment. Filtering doesn't flavor your water, but it can be time-consuming to filter water.
- **Ultraviolet light purifier (e.g., SteriPEN):** Ultraviolet light damages the DNA of all microorganisms, rendering them harmless. Water must be clear for the ultraviolet light to function, so all silt must be filtered before purification.
- **Boiling:** Boiling kills all microorganisms but is very time-consuming, requires a stove and fuel, and is not practical for dayhikers. A rolling boil should be established for one minute before consumption. Water does not need to be filtered before boiling.

See www.nps.gov/grca/planyourvisit/safe-water.htm for recommendations developed by the Grand Canyon National Park.

## Altitude Sickness

Altitude sickness is caused by hypoxia, the insufficient supply of oxygen to the body's tissues. At the South Rim of the Grand Canyon, elevation 7000 feet, there is approximately 80 percent as much oxygen as at sea level. At this elevation the serious forms of altitude sickness are not a concern. Instead, most people will notice they are at higher elevations only because they will become out of breath more easily and need to slow their pace. Above an elevation of 5000 feet, most individuals begin to show a decrease in cardiovascular capacity—approximately 10 percent for each 3000 feet climbed. If you are exercising hard and therefore approaching your maximum cardiovascular capacity, decrease your pace to avoid overexerting yourself.

## PREVENTING COMMON TRAIL HAZARDS

| HAZARD | PREVENTION |
|---|---|
| Hyponatremia | • Eat lots of salty snacks. |
| Dehydration | • Drink at least four liters of water per day. |
| Heat exhaustion and heatstroke | • Take breaks in the shade or lying in a creek.<br>• Wet your clothes at taps, in streams, or with a sprayer.<br>• Fan yourself. |
| Hypothermia | • During the cooler months, always carry warm, non-cotton clothes. |
| Falling | • Use trekking poles.<br>• Go slowly. |
| Blisters | • Wear broken-in, sturdy shoes or boots.<br>• Apply sports tape to potential hot spots before the hike.<br>• Stop and patch hot spots as soon as you feel them. |
| Flash floods | • Stay clear of obvious gullies during heavy rainfall, including the wash above Indian Garden and banks of Pipe Creek. |
| Lightning | • Avoid rim vistas.<br>• Don't dawdle on the upper stretches of the South Kaibab Trail. |
| Scorpions | • Shake out your clothes and shoes before getting dressed.<br>• Wear shoes in camp. |
| Waterborne pests | • Drink water from the taps or filter and purify your water. |
| Altitude sickness | • Go slowly, take breaks, drink plenty of water, and eat regularly. |
| Drowning in the Colorado | • Don't swim in the river. |

In addition, you may begin to feel the symptoms of Acute Mountain Sickness (AMS), defined as a collection of symptoms experienced while at "high" elevation, including a headache combined with one or more of the following: loss of appetite, nausea, vomiting, fatigue or weakness, dizziness or light-headedness, and difficulty sleeping. By definition AMS occurs above 7000 feet, but some people may feel symptoms at lower elevations.

To minimize your risk of altitude sickness, stay well hydrated and well fed, and don't push yourself too hard at the highest elevations. Keep in mind that even very fit people get altitude sickness. Also, remember that you are already pushing your body hard; this exertion combined with the high elevation can make you more vulnerable to heat exhaustion and heatstroke.

If you get a headache as you ascend, aspirin or ibuprofen will help relieve the symptoms, although many people prefer ibuprofen because it is effective in smaller doses. If taking an anti-inflammatory makes you feel better, you will also tend to eat and drink more, which may further minimize altitude sickness.

## Drowning in the Colorado

As a hiker there is no need to endanger yourself by swimming in the Colorado River. On a hot summer day its cool waters can be very enticing, but avoid the temptation. The water may appear smooth and harmless, but the current is deceptively strong. In recent decades more people have died while swimming in the river than while boating down it. Moreover, a disproportionate number of drowning deaths are hikers between the Bright Angel Campground and the mouth of Pipe Creek, who ignore the posted warnings to stay out of the water.

Cool yourself in the quiet waters of Bright Angel Creek or content yourself with wading to knee depth at the boat beach just upstream of Bright Angel Creek. Do not go for a dip at the mouth of Pipe Creek, an especially dangerous location, as Pipe Creek Rapids begin just downstream.

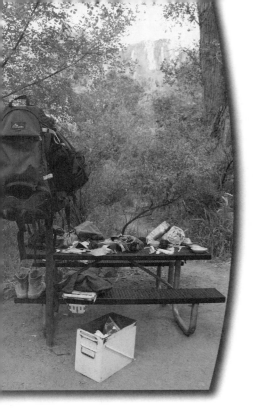

## 3
# Preparations and Planning

**B**ecause of permit quotas, the decision to camp inside the Grand Canyon cannot (usually) be spontaneous. Instead, you must begin the process of applying for an overnight permit more than four months in advance. This time delay, although frustrating if you like having flexibility, means that you have ample time to make sure you are planning exactly the hike you wish to take and are well prepared to make it a success. Dayhikers do not require a permit and can therefore make a spur-of-the-moment decision to descend. And if you haven't planned ahead, a few last-minute permits are available—keep reading.

## Choosing an Itinerary

A glance at a map of the Grand Canyon indicates that numerous trails descend to the Colorado River. However, only the three corridor trails—the Bright Angel, South Kaibab, and North Kaibab

*Above:* Food lockers, a backpack pole, and a picnic table are present at each campsite in the corridor trail campgrounds.

trails—are maintained to a "high" standard, indicating a more moderate grade, a wider trail that is generally easy to follow and walk along, and that the trails mostly have piped water, bathrooms, and emergency phones along their length. The National Park Service recommends that first time Grand Canyon visitors begin by backpacking along one of them.

This book further simplifies your decision-making, by focusing on (and recommending) a single loop that can be hiked in either direction: down the South Kaibab Trail and up the Bright Angel Trail or vice versa. The total distance is 16.1 miles. Either direction will result in you camping along the Colorado River at the Bright Angel Campground at the mouth of Bright Angel Creek and possibly at the Indian Garden Campground halfway up the Bright Angel Trail. (Dayhiking with a detour to the Bright Angel Campground for water cuts 0.4 mile from the distance. Dayhiking and taking the

## WHY DIDN'T YOU INCLUDE THE NORTH KAIBAB?

The North Kaibab Trail is also a beautiful, highly recommended route, but the South Kaibab to Bright Angel circuit is the *one best hike* in the Grand Canyon—you descend a ridge with exquisite views of the canyon, spend a night along the Colorado River, traipse along the River Trail for 2 miles to the start of the Bright Angel Trail, and ascend along Pipe Creek, Garden Creek, and a steep amphitheater made passable by the Bright Angel Fault. For the people who question my decision that this is a more classic hike than a rim-to-rim trip, I have two thoughts. First, while hiking the South Kaibab and Bright Angel trails, there are many points where you have a view down to the Colorado River and broad vistas across the canyon, continually reminding you that you are descending to the bottom of the Grand Canyon. My favorite aspect of the North Kaibab Trail is the scenery right next to you: the Pinnacles, Ribbon Falls, the Box, but not that wonderful feeling of plunging to the Colorado River. Second, a book titled "One Best Hike" doesn't suggest that there is *only* one good hike—this route is simply the best place to begin your Grand Canyon explorations.

River Trail, cuts 0.8 mile from your distance. The latter is not recommended, since you must carry sufficient water from the canyon rim to reach Indian Garden.)

Overall, I recommend a three- to four-day trip, descending the South Kaibab Trail, spending two nights at the Bright Angel Campground, and ascending the Bright Angel Trail. If time permits or you feel you need to split the ascent over two days, spend a night at Indian Garden and take a side trip to Plateau Point. Of course if you have only two free days, by all means descend one day and head back up the next. The trail descriptions are written assuming you descend the South Kaibab and ascend the Bright Angel, but since the text is divided into short trail segments, you can easily reserve the order you read the sections.

Some considerations you might use to select your exact itinerary are:

- **Semiloop or out-and-back:** You see twice as much trail during a loop hike as an out-and-back hike—a benefit of course. However, some people will choose to take the Bright Angel Trail both directions, due to the increased shade, availability of water, and the option of spending a night at Indian Garden on both the descent and ascent. Indeed, if a out-and-back hike suits you better, remember that the landscape looks very different when you are facing the opposite direction.
- **The view:** The most expansive views are from the South Kaibab Trail. However, the feeling of being in an amphitheater along the Bright Angel Trail is equally grand. And the upper miles of the Bright Angel Trail have excellent views across the canyon.
- **Availability of water:** The upper stretches of the Bright Angel Trail have purified water available for hikers. Water is unavailable on the South Kaibab Trail.
- **Steepness:** The South Kaibab Trail is the steeper of the choices, with stretches descending at a steady rate of 1000 feet per mile. It is therefore hardest on your knees while descending and your

*HINT: If you have time, plan a leisurely itinerary with an extra night at Bright Angel Campground and/or a night at Indian Garden Campground to have a chance to take side trips—or rest if you underestimated the endurance the hike requires. Possible side trips include Phantom Overlook, Ribbon Falls, Phantom Creek, and Plateau Point (see page 153).*

calves while ascending. However, most sections of both trails have a grade of approximately 700 feet per mile.

- **Multiple days for the ascent:** A 4600-foot ascent in a single day while carrying a backpack makes for a long, difficult day. Many people split the climb over two days, spending a night at Indian Garden Campground on the Bright Angel Trail. There are no camping options along the South Kaibab Trail—it must be done in one shot. (You could of course also spend an extra day at Indian Garden on your descent.)
- **Layover days:** If time permits, a layover day at the Bright Angel Campground affords the possibility of visiting Phantom Overlook (on the Clear Creek Trail), Ribbon Falls (on the North Kaibab Trail), or the Box (the narrow stretch of canyon on the North Kaibab Trail). If you have a free afternoon at Indian Garden, head out to Plateau Point to watch the sunset. (See page 153 for details of these side hikes.)

# When to Go

The trails descending from the South Rim of the Grand Canyon can be hiked year-round. And they are, for permits to camp at the Bright Angel Campground are nearly fully booked year-round—with an occasional spare slot midsummer or in winter.

However, the climate information on page 48 indicates your experience will vary greatly across the year. Most people's foremost consideration is avoiding or learning how to endure the sizzling temperatures in the Inner Gorge during the summer months (mid-May through mid-September, and especially June through August), but day length, the possibility of icy trails just below the rim, overly cold temperatures, rainfall, and the chance to enjoy wildflowers may also influence your decision.

Most people consider spring (mid-March through April) or fall (late September through October) the preferred time for a visit. During these seasons, you are unlikely to experience freezing temperatures below 4000 feet (the elevation of the Indian Garden Campground) and the Inner Gorge will not be uncomfortably hot. These are also the driest months (see page 48), when winter storms and afternoon thundershowers are less likely to interfere with your adventure. In April or May you may be treated to a beautiful display of wildflowers. Spring and fall are the most difficult times of year to get overnight permits, and they're the only times it is somewhat sensible to dayhike, as temperatures are less extreme.

In winter, expect chilly temperatures during the morning and evening hours, especially if you camp at Indian Garden. You will need to navigate icy sections of trail, especially the top of the Bright Angel Trail and the first switchbacks on the South Kaibab Trail. The air will be cool and crisp and the sun's low angle produces both beautiful lighting and lots of shadows. And, while the backcountry campgrounds may still be full, you will encounter far fewer dayhikers on your journey and have more solitude. Dayhiking is not recommended, for although you can hike throughout the day, you do not want to be approaching the upper, icy sections of trail while exhausted, much less in the dark. Instead of heat exhaustion, you are vulnerable to hypothermia.

I usually avoid the desert during the summer months, but the land is still beautiful and captivating—the extreme climate can even be enticing. And of course this is vacation time and maybe your only chance to visit the Grand Canyon. During summer, start hiking by dawn, so that you can climb above the Inner Gorge before the sun climbs far into the sky. During these months, you are likely to choose to exit via the Bright Angel Trail and spend midday

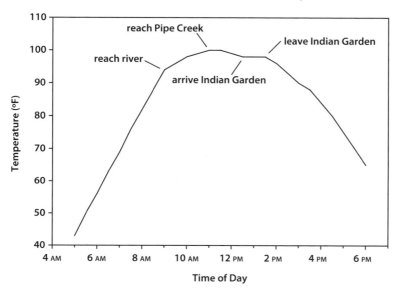

**Temperatures to Expect on a Mid-June Dayhike**

planted in the shade of Indian Garden, continuing upward only in the late afternoon. The extreme temperatures make dayhiking very impractical in summer, since you will want to avoid the Inner Gorge from quite early in the morning until the sun is setting, leaving insufficient daylight to climb back to the rim. Consider the figure (previous page), showing possible temperatures you will encounter in mid-June, if you require 12 hours hiking time, an additional hourlong lunch break, and leave at 5 A.M.

## Wilderness Permits

Permits are required for anyone camping below the canyon rim overnight, but not for dayhikes and stays at Phantom Ranch (see page 81 for more about the ranch). Only 10 percent of permits are available first-come, first-served at the Backcountry Information Center, so it is best to reserve your permit, as described below.

Backcountry camping regulations are quite different for the three corridor trails (those described in this book and the North Kaibab Trail) versus other regions in the backcountry; along the corridor trails, camping is permitted only in the three established campgrounds: Indian Garden, Bright Angel, and Cottonwood. (The rest of the park is divided into "use areas" with "at large" camping.)

*HINT: You must reserve a specific campground, but not campsite, for each night when you request a permit. You select your campsite when you arrive at the campground.*

Each of these campgrounds has specific campsites, some explicitly for small groups (1–6 people) and others for large groups (7–11 people). The table below shows the breakdown of sites at each campground. One group of the appropriate size is allowed at each campsite. In addition, there is a maximum number of people allowed in the campground each night, and that number indicates that all campsites cannot be filled to capacity each night—indeed many will be filled with small parties. Overall, smaller groups have a better chance at procuring a site.

| Campground | Small Group Sites | Large Group Sites | Maximum People |
|---|---|---|---|
| Indian Garden | 15 | 1 | 45 |
| Bright Angel | 31 | 2 | 90 |

From March 1 until November 14, a group may spend only two nights at each campsite (consecutive or nonconsecutive) per trip. It is illegal for a large group to split into subgroups to get multiple permits for the same campground for the same night. This regulation was a response to large groups of Boy Scouts camping in many adjacent campsites but functioning as a "single" group.

## PERMIT RESERVATIONS

Permits can be *requested* from the Grand Canyon National Park Backcountry Information Center beginning on the first of the month, four months before your entry date. For instance, requests for the month of March begin on the previous November 1 and requests for the month of October begin on June 1. You can download the permit request form from the overnight hiking and backcountry permit section of the park's website: www.nps.gov/grca/planyourvisit/overnight-hiking.htm.

Submit this form in one of three ways:

1. **Fax** your request to: Backcountry Information Center, 928-638-2125.
2. **Mail** your request to: Backcountry Information Center, P.O. Box 129, Grand Canyon, AZ 86023
3. **Hand deliver** your request to the Backcountry Information Center.

On your permit request form, list acceptable alternative dates and itineraries. Being flexible increases your likelihood of receiving a permit. At times of the year, especially October, the most popular month, the park may receive up to three times as many permit requests as they have slots.

If your request is successful, your permit and a CD titled *Hiking Grand Canyon* will be sent to you in the mail within a month. The permit you receive in the mail is all you need to embark on your walk; you do not need to visit the Backcountry Information Center before beginning your descent. The content from the CD, as well as podcasts and videos on all

*HINT: Permits* **received by 5** P.M. *on the first day of a given month are processed randomly. Permits received on subsequent days are processed in the order they are received. Since mailed permit requests cannot be postmarked until the first of the month, faxing (or hand delivering) your permit request gives you an enormous advantage.*

manner of Grand Canyon topics, are available on the multimedia section of the National Park Service website: www.nps.gov/grca/photosmultimedia/grca_pod.htm. For additional information, you can also call the Backcountry Information Center at 928-638-7875 between 1 P.M. and 5 P.M.

## LAST-MINUTE PERMITS

Approximately 10 percent of permits can be obtained first-come, first-served at the Backcountry Information Center. To obtain these permits, show up on a given morning before 8 A.M. During popular hiking seasons (almost always!), you will be assigned a number. At 8 A.M., the rangers call hikers up in numerical order and begin issuing permits for the *next* day. If the permit you request is not available, you can select a different hike, get a new number for the next morning, or give up. The new number you receive will be smaller, since some of the people ahead will likely have obtained a permit and others run out of time and headed home. If you have many days, you will probably get a permit eventually, but if you have only a few days you may very well end up empty-handed, especially if you wish to hike the corridor trails.

This method can be especially frustrating, for even if you have spare time for dayhikes, you can never start a dayhike until well after 8 A.M. Moreover, there might never be permits for the day you want, since groups might have shown up several days earlier and claimed the first-come, first-served sites for a whole string of days.

*HINT: Once you have received your permit in the mail, promptly reserve a nearby campsite or hotel for the nights before and after your hike. See page 108 for information.*

There is a little quirk in what is happening at the Backcountry Information Center each morning, especially at the end of the month. In addition to the people waiting to get the unreserved permits, a line of locals (including local guide services) wait until the first of the month to turn in their reservation requests; by handing them over in person first thing in the morning, they are virtually assured of the trip itinerary they want.

## FEES

Regardless of how you get your wilderness permit, there are fees. The permit itself costs $10. (This fee is waived if you purchase a

## ASSIGNING PERMITS

Assigning permits is a difficult—and currently noncomputerized—task for the rangers. They look at each permit request form to ensure that: 1) the group can realistically travel between the use zones or campsites they have requested, 2) multiple groups traveling in different directions do not all converge in a single use area on a given night, and 3) a group doesn't "hog" campsites. As they scrutinize each application, they may slightly adjust requested itineraries to match availability. And rangers have indicated that if you request backpacking permits for a rim-to-rim-to-rim trip, you might only receive half of your request, to make space for other people.

yearly $25 frequent hiker membership.) In addition there is a $5 per person per night fee. These fees apply both for reserved and first-come, first-served permits.

# Staying at Phantom Ranch

Not everyone who "backpacks" into the Grand Canyon stays at the Bright Angel Campground; some stay at Phantom Ranch, the backcountry lodge just upstream of the campground (see page 11 for the long history of this beautiful location). Some guests at the ranch arrive on mules, but many others hike down themselves. Phantom Ranch guests need to carry only a daypack; a bed and served meals await them at the ranch, making it an excellent choice if you want to spend a night in the Grand Canyon but are hesitant about camping or carrying a large pack. The 11 private cabins and 4 dormitory bunkhouses can accommodate 92 people, with the private cabins generally allocated to visitors arriving on mules. Reservations are taken 13 months in advance.

Phantom Ranch offers other services that may be tempting for campers. Quite a few campers traipse up to Phantom Ranch for one or more of their meals (breakfast, sack lunch, and your choice of a steak dinner or the hiker's stew). In addition they offer a duffle service: Up to 30 pounds of your gear descends on a mule, while you walk.

See www.grandcanyonlodges.com/lodging-704.html for rates and additional information.

# Training

Once you have your coveted backcountry permit, you must begin preparing for your hike. As you train, remember you are training to ensure you reach the river, return unaided to the rim, and *have a good time in the process.* After all, an odd corollary of "descending first" (see page 84) is that there is a high success rate; most people who decide to hike to the Colorado River reach their goal. But it also means that there are a lot of overextended people attempting to extricate themselves from the canyon—it is especially essential to be adequately conditioned, physically and mentally, for your adventure.

## PHYSICAL TRAINING

You need to be in sufficiently good physical condition that you can cover the necessary distance on downhill and uphill trails. To successfully hike to the bottom of the Grand Canyon and back up again, you will need to be able to hike at least 6 miles carrying a pack on three consecutive days, climb 4500 feet (over one to two days, depending on your route and itinerary), and tolerate dry and hot (or cold) conditions.

Any aerobic exercise will help you get in shape, but the muscles used extensively for walking down and up hills can really be conditioned only by walking down and up hills. If you live somewhere with hills, the best form of training is, unsurprisingly, to take long walks. However, if your surroundings are flatter, or you don't have time to hike hills regularly, cities are full of training opportunities: Walk up and down staircases in a tall building, walk up and down bleachers in a local stadium, or use a stair machine at a gym. Do not underestimate the descent into the canyon; sore muscles and most importantly, knee injuries are less likely if the muscles you need to descend gracefully are strong.

Testing your endurance ahead of time ensures that you are physically and mentally ready to walk for many hours. If you are able to complete a 10-mile hike in hilly terrain, you are physically capable of a multiday trip. If you plan to approach it as a dayhike, you should be able to hike 15 miles in hilly terrain stopping for only 10 minutes each hour, plus a couple longer "lunch" breaks.

An added reason for training hikes is to break in a pair of hiking boots or shoes (see more on footwear on page 93). You will better be able to enjoy your hike out of the canyon if you're not focused on painful feet.

## MENTAL PREPARATION

In addition to physical training, there are two mental challenges, both very important and in slight opposition to one another. The first is knowing how your body performs in both "easy" and adverse environmental conditions and understanding "messages" your body sends. To avoid many of the conditions described in Precautions and Considerations (see page 53), you should be familiar with how you feel when you are simply tired, so you can recognize symptoms not attributed to your normal exhaustion. The ability to perceive when your body no longer feels "good" or "normal" can only be gained by exercising frequently and paying attention to your body. You should be especially attentive to your body's warning signs if you have a history of heart problems or if you were relatively inactive until the inspiration to backpack the Grand Canyon grabbed you. Quite a few people—especially men in their 50s and 60s—die of cardiac arrest on these trails, probably because they pushed themselves too hard in the hot, dry conditions.

The second mental challenge is finding the motivation to keep moving toward your destination when you are tired. If you have read about all the possible dangers waiting to befall you, you may be convinced that if you are tired on a hot day, you should hide in the shade, but it is important to know the difference between "tired" and "body malfunctioning"—almost everyone hiking up 4500 feet will be tired. And all those tired people need to take the recommended breaks (see page 88) and then keep hauling themselves up the hill at a steady pace. The mental games required to motivate yourself to continue are individualistic, and determining the right pace for your body can only be established through practice hikes (see page 85 for more about pacing yourself).

## ACCLIMATIZING TO DESERT HEAT

Heat acclimatization is a very important part of preparing to hike in the Grand Canyon during the hot months. Only people who live in an equally hot environment can truly acclimatize to the heat, as complete acclimatization requires two to three weeks of daily (or near daily) exercise in hot conditions. Physiologically, heat acclimatization includes increased sweating, increased blood volume, increased blood flow to the skin (which promotes cooling), and increased water intake.

However, limited heat acclimatization occurs after only four to seven days, so visitors from cooler climes can acclimatize by scheduling their Grand Canyon descent for the end of a Southwest vacation. First spend at least a week visiting and taking shorter hikes in nearby—and equally hot—national parks, to acclimatize to the desert climate.

# What to Contemplate Before Descending

By the time you reach Grand Canyon Village, you will have spent many hours planning, training, and assembling your gear. This section covers a few more considerations: reminders about pace, breaks, group dynamics, and what it means to descend first—topics to read about before you leave home and to have firmly etched in your mind during your hike. For each of these I can provide advice but no tangible rules. How you implement these suggestions is affected by individualistic factors: what pace and break schedule works best for you and your judgment and attitudes about pushing yourself, safety, and group etiquette.

### DESCENDING FIRST, ASCENDING SECOND

The National Park Service at the Grand Canyon is very insistent that hiking the Grand Canyon is much more strenuous than most people expect it to be—and they are correct. Most likely, on the majority of steep hikes you have taken you have parked your car at a relatively low elevation and begun your day with an ascent. Canyons turn everything upside down: You begin by going downhill and then have to complete the arduous ascent. Think about what this means:

- **The descent is optional. Going up isn't.** Most people can rapidly descend many thousands of feet—indeed most people can effortlessly descend far more elevation than they can easily regain, especially later the same day. If you are climbing a mountain and you run out of energy on the ascent, you are quite likely to be able to turn around and descend without much trouble. But what do you do if getting to the top isn't optional? In the Grand Canyon, every last person who begins the ascent from the bottom **must reach the summit**. You must be very aware of your capabilities—especially if attempting a long dayhike—before descending.

- **Take care of yourself on the descent.** On the descent from a mountain summit, it is advisable to take breaks and take it easy; if you push yourself, you will pay for it by being unnecessarily exhausted that evening and having very sore muscles the next day. If you do not take care of your body on your descent into the Grand Canyon, you will have a much harder time on the ascent. Take it easy on the descent: Walk at a moderate pace, take breaks, and stay well fed and hydrated.

- **You will be at the highest elevations at the end of the day** when you are already exhausted. The 7000-foot South Rim isn't all that high, but having 20 percent less oxygen than usual makes the ascent a bit harder.

- **As a dayhiker, you experience the hottest temperatures as you begin your ascent.** Instead of climbing to higher, and cooler, elevations as the day progresses, you spend the cool morning at high elevation and the sizzling midday at low elevations. In summer a dayhiker can escape the inner canyon midday (and even midmorning) heat only by descending the entire route predawn, which quite honestly seems a little pointless. In spring and fall, beginning to descend slightly before dawn may be sufficient for a fast, well-trained hiker.

## PACE

If you manage to establish and maintain an appropriate pace for this hike, you will have greater endurance and find the walking much more enjoyable. Although this advice is given often, only considerable hiking experience in similar conditions will help you fine-tune your exact pace. I have learned that a range of paces feel "good" to me, but if I have to move more quickly, I need far too many breaks and my legs get tired prematurely. Alternately, if I hike more slowly than my normal pace, my legs and breathing never settle into a sustainable rhythm, and both my endurance and motivation are much reduced. For this reason some groups may decide it is OK for the faster hikers to go ahead and then take longer rests every few miles, allowing everyone to regroup.

Think about your choice of pace even while walking downhill. It is very easy to race downhill when you are fresh, oblivious to the fact that you are expending calories, using your muscles, baking in the sun, and pounding your feet. However, you will need energy, muscles, and functional feet for the ascent and should slow your pace to more of a plod than a brisk walk—absolutely essential if you are attempting a long dayhike, but still true if you are spending a night along the river because sore muscles and feet will not heal overnight.

On the ascent, remember the old mantra that *slow and steady wins the race.* Or rephrase this to *slower* and steady wins the race. At the bottom of a long climb, whatever pace I can do, going a little slower and having a steadier pace will get me up most efficiently. Observations and experience have taught me that most people start up a hill at a pace too fast to sustain for long. You should actually go more slowly than your "sustainable" pace for the first half mile to mile, because your muscles need some time to warm up.

On your training hikes, you can identify your ideal range of paces. Try different walking paces on different days, to learn how your lungs and legs feel under different conditions. Over time you will discover a pace that feels good. There are two tricks to converting that knowledge into a successful hike into and out of the Grand Canyon. First, take enough training hikes so that you know exactly how your lungs and legs feel when your pace is sustainable for a long climb, rather than how fast you were going on a given day. After all, the actual distance covered and elevation gained per time can be wildly different on different trails and at different temperatures, but you'll have the same pairs of legs and lungs. Second, on a very long hike, such as this, force yourself to go about 80 percent of your good pace. I have hiked with many very fit, gung-ho hikers who sped past me during the first hours of the walk, but ran out of reserves long before the top and ended up dragging.

Ingrain in your mind that neither backpackers nor dayhikers need to hike quickly to complete this hike. The distance from Bright Angel Campground to the South Rim via the Bright Angel Trail is 9.3 miles and the distance down and up is 16.1 miles. A backpacker, given an early start, will have ample time. A dayhiker should average about 1.5 miles per hour. These are steady plodding paces!

Members of a group will likely modify their paces somewhat to stick together. While it is appropriate for fast walkers to slow down, slow walkers should not feel obliged to quicken their pace; that approach is more likely to lead to a much slower pace or even medical problems before the end of the day.

## GROUP DYNAMICS

When group members have different expectations, a hike is more likely to be remembered as unsuccessful—either because it was aborted or you harbor negative memories. Even if your companions are regular hiking partners, discuss goals and hiking styles before beginning your descent. Topics for discussion include:

- If you are planning a hike, consider whether you prefer to hike alone or as part of a group. Hiking alone gives you much more flexibility: You get to set your own pace, take breaks when you wish, and pick a departure time that suits you. You also get to enjoy the canyon's grandeur in solitude. However, traveling alone reduces your safety margin, and for many people, the camaraderie of their hiking partners is an important part of their backpacking experience.
- If you are part of a group, discuss before the hike whether group members should stick together or hike at their own paces. If all group members are comfortable with the group being dispersed, members of a party do not need to stick together while hiking on a trail. However, everyone should be carrying a map, and the group should agree on meeting points every mile or two, including all trail junctions. It is absolutely essential that *all* party members study the maps together and *all* know where the next meeting point is. Pick well-known, well-labeled meeting points, such as the resthouses, Indian Garden, mouth of Pipe Creek, or the Tipoff. Another option is for a strong hiker to remain at the back of the group, take a longer break, and catch up with other party members along the way. *If any group members find themselves overexerted, struggling with the heat, questioning their ability to be alone, or sick, everyone needs to stick together, to aid and encourage each other.*
- Members of a group should agree in advance whether it is acceptable for the most energetic members to take extra excursions, such as a late afternoon jaunt up to Phantom Overlook or Plateau Point, on their own.
- Agree upon your departure time the night before, especially for a midsummer, predawn start from Bright Angel

Campground. If you know you are slow getting ready in the morning, get up a little earlier. Your hiking companions will become increasingly frustrated if they sit around camp for half an hour feeling the temperature rise.

## BREAKS

While it is important to establish that *slower and steady* pace that propels you to the canyon rim, you should still take many breaks on your ascent. Your breaks should include quick breathers, drink breaks, 10-minute food and rest breaks each hour, and longer rest breaks a few times during your ascent, especially if you are hiking on a hot day.

The shortest breaks are quick breathers—all but the best-trained individuals will need a few of these on the steeper sections. You will also want to take 30-second water stops every five to ten minutes, either to gulp water from your hydration tube or to grab that handy bottle of water and slurp some down. But be careful not to let these half-minute breaks take up more than that; you don't want your leg muscles to cool down or to lose the good walking rhythm you have established.

Next, take a ten-minute break each hour to refuel on food, drink extra water, and patch blisters, if possible in a shady spot, such as at the resthouses, at Indian Garden, under the rock overhang in the Tapeats Narrows along Garden Creek, under a pinyon at Cedar Ridge, or any other little spot you can find. If you are the fastest member of a group, remember that the break begins, not ends, when the last person arrives. Make sure the stragglers also get 10 minutes to rest their legs and eat some food. If you are antsy to get going, pull out this book and read about the area's geology and vegetation.

Finally, most individuals will take one or two longer breaks for lunch or a midafternoon siesta. If you are ascending midsummer, take a much longer midday break in the shade of Indian Garden, to minimize hiking between the hours of 10 A.M. and 4 P.M.

## DAYHIKING

As described in the introduction, this book is aimed at hikers spending two or more days completing their descent into and ascent from the Grand Canyon—both because the National Park Service strongly urges people not to complete the hike in a day and because you miss a lot of the experience when hiking at the fast, often rushed pace of a dayhiker or trail runner. This is a **location hike**, in contrast to a **destination hike** (see page 3 for an explanation), meaning that this is not a hike where most people's most gratifying moment is crossing the Colorado River, but where they will be equally awed by the experience at many points along the way. The first time I hiked the South Kaibab and Bright Angel loop was as a very quickly paced dayhike. Although I have an uncanny ability to remember most hikes I've taken nearly step by step, when I revisited the trails some years later, I realized I *barely* remembered the scenery. I'd pushed myself too hard to take it in.

With that preamble, my brief counts on the trail suggest that during all but the hottest and coldest months, people dayhiking to the Colorado River *outnumber* people backpacking. Most of these people clearly hike a lot, are in very good shape, and many are very used to desert conditions. If you're not sure you fit into **all three** of these categories, think hard about following the park service's recommendations of dayhiking no farther than Plateau Point on the Bright Angel Trail. If you know you fit into these categories, you have only a day (or no permit), and the high temperature at Phantom Ranch is supposed to be less than 85°F, you could attempt this endurance test.

If you decide to descend and ascend the entire canyon, read the summary table of how to avoid hazards (page 71), carry plenty of water, eat plenty of food, and take frequent breaks, even on the way down.

# Familiarizing Yourself with the Landscape

In addition to acclimatizing to the heat (see page 83), arriving at the Grand Canyon a few days before the start of your hike lets you become familiar with the landscape. Staring down on the Bright Angel and South Kaibab trails before you descend helps put your hike in perspective. You can see the big picture more clearly while on the rim. Go to Trailview Overlook or Yavapai Point (and the adjacent visitor center) to see where these two trails descend through the rock layers. Take note of how the Bright Angel Trail descends a broad gully, the Bright Angel Fault line (see page 21 for more about geology and trail location). Notice how the distance from the South Rim to the Colorado River is shorter than from the

North Rim to the bottom, a consequence of streams on the South Rim flowing away from the canyon and those on the North Rim flowing to the canyon (see more about the rim elevations on page 25). The Grand Canyon is overwhelming—in the most wonderful way—and having a day or two to enjoy it before you put on a big pack will enhance your hike.

# What to Bring

The water, food, first-aid kit, and other essentials you carry to the Colorado River and back ensure that you have a safe and enjoyable journey. Deciding what is required is a delicate balance between being encumbered by an excessively heavy backpack and neglecting to bring the required items. My basic rule is to carry sufficient gear to spend an unplanned night on the trail. Most importantly, that means you must always be carrying several liters of water, while in winter a dayhiker must also have sufficient clothing to sit through a very cold night.

I have divided my recommendations on what to pack into water, food, footwear, the 10 essentials, additional gear for a dayhike, and additional gear for a backpacking trip. (Backpackers will need to read through all lists, but can omit a daypack.) A checklist of the items in each of the sections is provided on page 102.

## WATER

Consuming sufficient water and food—and in the proper ratio is difficult for many people, especially if the heat, dry air, or simply exertion makes eating unappealing. Dehydration, caused by drinking less water than you are losing through sweating, breathing, and urination, is one problem. Hyponatremia, or having too few salts (specifically sodium) in your blood, is a second problem, and actually the greater risk while hiking in the Grand Canyon. Hyponatremia is caused by drinking copious quantities of water and can be exacerbated by eating insufficient food. After all, the dry desert air and exertion make people thirsty, and as long as water is available, most people will drink regularly. If you are hot and tired, however, it is much more difficult to remember to stop and eat.

To consume sufficient water on your hike, you must carry and drink enough. The first requires planning in any desert environment, since water is available in limited locations. While most Grand Canyon hikes require hikers to carry water for the entire day, purified water is available along the Bright Angel Trail, allowing you to refill at several locations: 1.5-Mile Resthouse, 3-Mile Resthouse, and Indian Garden. Purified water is also available at the Bright Angel Campground, including a tap a little west of the lower campground bridge. The latter is useful knowledge if you are dayhiking and wish to take the shortest detour from the River Trail. (Note that water is not available at the 1.5-Mile and 3-Mile resthouses during the winter months. Ask the rangers about water availability before beginning your hike.) If you plan to get water from side streams or the Colorado River, you will need to treat or filter it (see page 69 for a description of possible devices).

*HINT: At each break I check my water supply and make sure it is disappearing at the rate of a quart every 2 to 3 miles.*

To ensure you have sufficient water to reach the next tap, you should have enough container(s) to carry at least 3 liters—a gallon if you plan to ascend the South Kaibab Trail. Either carry it in water bottles or use a bladder-and-tube hydration system. Carrying a water bottle lets you efficiently gulp large quantities of water, but you need to be disciplined enough to stop frequently to drink. Alternatively, a bladder-and-tube hydration system allows you to drink as you are walking, letting you slowly and steadily consume water throughout your hike. I recommend the latter: I nearly doubled my water consumption when I switched to this system, because I drank a few sips every five minutes, whereas I'd previously procrastinated about taking out my water bottle until I was really thirsty, once every half hour at best. If you use a bladder-and-tube hydration system, carry a liter of spare water in a bottle in case you are too efficient at drinking water and don't realize you are running out.

About 5 to 8 quarts of water should be adequate for most people on a full day-hike. If you are hiking more than eight hours, this suggestion is lower than the oft-stated "drink a quart an hour," but research on soldiers exerting themselves in desert environments indicates that, even with all-day exertion, 8 quarts a day is adequate. (If you feel like your body needs more water than this, limit the

*HINT: On a winter hike you still need to consume quite a bit of water, but are less inclined to drink cold water on a cold day. Bring a thermos of warm tea or electrolyte mix (many of which taste quite good warm) or fill your water containers with warm water.*

number of hours you are active, especially if you are not well acclimatized to desert conditions.)

## FOOD

On a two-day trip descending to the Colorado River and climbing back to the South Rim with a moderately sized backpack, you will expend somewhere in the vicinity of 8,000 calories. A dayhiker will expend about 5,000. Although you are unlikely to replenish all calories consumed—after all part of the joy of hiking is weighing less at the end of your trip—carry at least 3,000 calories per day and eat throughout the day.

Both dayhikers and overnight hikers should eat a 200- to 500-calorie snack (or "lunch") every hour or two. Eat plenty of salty foods, such as salted nuts, chips, or jerky. Energy bars, granola bars, dried fruit, and cookies also make excellent snacks. Easily digestible snacks, like Gu, provide your body with an easily accessible supply of energy and are also generally still appealing when you are exhausted. I always bring one larger "snack" (bread or crackers with toppings) that I call lunch and eat as I take a longer midday break in the shade, but hearty snacks throughout the day provide sufficient calories and salts. It is a good idea to bring a variety of snack food and treats, so that you always find something appealing.

In addition to lunch and snacks, overnight hikers need to carry hearty breakfasts and dinners. Bring any lightweight, flavorful food that appeals to your palette. Instant oatmeal and granola with powdered milk are two backpacker breakfast favorites. Add a handful of dried fruit or nuts to your bowl for extra energy and flavor.

I always begin my dinners with a cup of instant soup. During cold-weather months it provides welcome warmth, and year-round it delivers an infusion of salt. For dinner itself, either freeze-dried backpacking meals or your own creations are good alternatives, but make sure the freeze-dried meals contain sufficient calories for you (they don't for me) and that your own creations are appealing—you have to eat. One of my favorite concoctions that includes all food groups and is very compact to carry is something I call "5-C couscous": couscous, curry powder, dried cranberries, cashews, and powdered coconut milk. Check your local

*HINT: Electrolyte drinks don't provide your body with sufficient salts or the correct balance of salts, and therefore should not be consumed in lieu of food. In particular, they contain little sodium.*

outdoor store for wilderness cuisine cookbooks. The store in Grand Canyon Village carries a good selection of freeze-dried backpacking meals.

Some hikers staying at Bright Angel Campground opt to eat breakfast and dinner at Phantom Ranch, eliminating the need to carry a camping stove and making their food bags much lighter. Their dinner stew is delicious! Once you have a backpacking permit, contact Phantom Ranch to determine their availability of "meals only" slots (see page 81 for more information).

## FOOTWEAR

Each person's feet (and ankles and knees) have different needs in footwear. The only consensus among people I've hiked with is to wear a pair of comfortable, well broken-in, but not worn-out shoes on a long hike. These shoes could be full leather hiking boots, lightweight cloth-and-leather hiking boots, trail runners, or lightweight running shoes. On trails in the Grand Canyon shoes with good tread are essential since sections of the trail have a surface deposit of small rocks overlying a layer of compacted soil, creating a slippery surface.

These few footwear suggestions should transcend the "lightweight" versus "lots of support" debate:

- If you wear trail runners, don't choose a pair with a tall, hiking boot-like platform; it elevates your foot above the ground and raises your foot's center of gravity. Since you do not have any ankle support, this design increases your chances of twisting an ankle and has no advantages.
- Don't wear old running shoes with worn-out padding. After 2,000 to 3,000 steps per mile in rugged terrain for 16 miles, any foot will feel sore in a worn-out shoe.
- Taping your heels before heading uphill will reduce the likelihood of blisters.
- Bring an extra pair of socks, even for a dayhike. If your feet start to feel beat up, switch to a clean pair of socks with not-yet-compressed padding to give your feet new life.
- Take your shoes off during extended breaks, giving your feet, socks, and shoes a chance to dry out.
- Wear a pair of ankle-high gaiters to keep pebbles and sand out of your shoes. Keeping the inside of your shoes clean reduces the likelihood of blisters.

- Bring a pair of trekking poles. They lessen the impact of your toes on your shoes during the descent and help your shoes keep traction, minimizing your chances of falling.

In the interest of full disclosure, I'm biased toward heavy hiking boots, which provide the ankle and foot support that I require. In lighter shoes, I end up with very sore feet. The downside is that I often get blisters, but I successfully combat them with multiple layers of sports tape, applied before I start walking. Many others prefer the discomfort of sore feet to hauling extra weight around, or their feet are content in lightweight shoes.

Only you can determine what pair of shoes is right for your feet. Experiment with different choices on your practice hikes, ensuring that they are comfortable in rocky terrain, uphill, downhill, when your feet are sweaty, and after many hours of walking. Moreover, if no pair of shoes is perfect—which is likely the case—after a few test walks, you will be aware of their shortcomings and be able to combat problems as they occur.

## TEN ESSENTIALS

Packing the 10 essentials is an excellent way to start organizing your gear for a long hike. As you place them in your pack, remind yourself why it is essential that you carry each of them. The official list is: map, compass, sunglasses and sunscreen, extra food and water (discussed above), extra clothes, headlamp or flashlight, first-aid kit, fire starter, matches, and a knife.

1. **Map:** Simply put, it is dangerous to enter the wilderness without a map. This warning is especially appropriate for hikers in the Grand Canyon, where contorted canyons and desert landscape can be particularly disorienting and appear repetitive, making it difficult to determine where you came from. The corridor trails in the Grand Canyon are well signed, but if you stray from the trail or mistakenly wander onto a different trail (such as the Tonto Trail), you need to determine where you are and how to navigate back to the trail.

    The maps in this book show the trail and some of the surrounding landscape, but their limited geographic extent will not help you relocate yourself if you deviate from the corridor trails. Trail maps of the entire national park produced by Trails Illustrated and Sky Terrain include a much greater area than you need, but they give you a good sense of the relative location of trails and landforms if you need to orient yourself. (While a GPS unit can provide the same information, it's a secondary navigation tool, since it runs on batteries, might stop working if dropped, and often picks up insufficient satellites near tall walls.)

2. **Compass:** The only time you are likely to use a compass is if you become lost and disoriented and need to orient your map, identify some basic landmarks, and thereby determine

## THE DIFFERENT TYPES OF SOLAR RADIATION

The wavelengths of interest to us that are emitted from the sun include visible light, heat, and ultraviolet (UV) rays. Of these, UV rays are the highest energy and therefore do the most damage your body. UV radiation is further divided into UVA, UVB, and UVC, of which UVA is the weakest and UVC the highest energy (and potentially most damaging). Each type attenuates differently in the atmosphere and affects our skin differently.

The atmosphere absorbs all of the UVC rays and most of the UVB rays, but little of the UVA. This distinction is accentuated in the early morning, late afternoon, and during the fall and winter months: When the sun is lower on the horizon, the rays pass through more atmosphere. As a result, a proportionally higher amount of UVB radiation is absorbed at a lower sun angle, meaning that UVB, but not UVA, shows considerable diurnal and seasonal variation.

The causes of skin cancer are an active field of research, but current evidence suggests that while UVB causes most sunburns (and is necessary for Vitamin D production), exposure to both UVB and UVA lead to skin cancer. In other words, you are much more likely to receive a painful sunburn during midday and midsummer (not to mention at high elevation where there is less atmosphere to absorb UV radiation), but are still subjecting yourself to skin cancer risk when the sun is low in the sky. And therefore, while it is tempting to apply sunscreen only when you are most likely to end up reddened, it is important to always apply sunscreen and/or wear long sleeves.

the direction to the trail or which direction to follow the trail. (Many GPS units do not include a compass.)

3. **Sunglasses and sunscreen:** As you descend into the Grand Canyon, you can only escape the sun under riparian trees, in rest shelters, against a tall rock wall or overhang, and maybe pressed tightly against the trunk of a pinyon or juniper tree. As you walk you must protect yourself from the sun with sunglasses, sunscreen, and a wide-brimmed hat. If you ignore these essentials, you could get more than a nasty burn; repeated exposure can lead to skin cancer and cataracts. Your sunscreen and sunglasses should protect you against both UVA and UVB, and your sunscreen should be at least SPF 30. To avoid chapped or split lips, bring lip balm that is at least SPF 15. Apply sunscreen every two to four hours during your hike—or as recommended on the sunscreen container—research indicates it becomes ineffective over time.

4. **Food:** See page 92.

5. **Water:** See page 90.

6. **Extra clothes:** Every hiker needs sufficient warm clothing to spend a night on the trail at any elevation. However, the type of clothing varies greatly by season. At one extreme, in winter,

## HOW MUCH DOES LIGHT-COLORED CLOTHING HELP?

It isn't just the outside temperature and the intensity of exercise that determines how hot you get. Solar radiation hitting you directly also increases your body temperature. On a hot, sunny day you, therefore, want to deflect as much of the solar radiation as possible. About half of solar radiation is in infrared wavelengths (what we sense as hot, but cannot see) and much of the rest is from visible wavelengths. Light-colored clothing reflects most of the visible wavelengths, but all standard clothing absorbs most of the infrared wavelengths. Aluminized fabrics and some specially coated fabrics reflect nearly all visible and infrared wavelengths, keeping you much cooler, but these are not widely available. A wide-brimmed hat does a fantastic job of keeping you cooler, since the brim prevents all radiation from hitting your skin and clothes and is not in direct contact with your skin, minimizing conductive heat transfer.

you should have thermal tops and bottoms, a warm hat, a fleece jacket, and a waterproof jacket at minimum, and probably gloves, fleece pants, waterproof pants, and a down vest or jacket. The Grand Canyon is chilly in winter. But even midsummer, nighttime temperature near the rim dip into the 40s. During the summer months complement the clothes you hike in (a shirt and shorts or hiking pants) with a thermal top and a windbreaker (or lightweight rain jacket if rain is forecast).

*HINT: Reduce your susceptibility to heatstroke by wearing light-colored, loose-fitting clothes and a wide-brimmed hat. Fabrics with tight weaves, such as synthetic fabrics with sun protection (UPF) ratings keep you cooler than loosely woven fabrics, like linen. One benefit of cotton is that if you wet it whenever you pass water, it holds more water to keep you cool through evaporative cooling.*

The backcountry rangers in the Grand Canyon report that in summer people wearing cotton clothing stay cooler than those wearing other fabrics, explaining that this is because water evaporates more slowly from cotton. I have a difficult time understanding the physics behind this recommendation, since the same amount of sweat evaporates through either, creating the same cooling effect. Maybe it applies only when you soak your clothes in water, since a cotton T-shirt holds more water?

7. **Headlamp or flashlight:** Backpackers will choose to carry a flashlight or headlamp for use around camp, but dayhikers should also include one in their packs so they can begin their hike predawn and (perhaps unintentionally) continue their hike after dark. Plus, in an emergency, a light can be used to attract the attention of other visitors.

The widely available light-emitting diode (LED) headlamps are so tiny, weigh only a few ounces, and continue to run on the same set of AAA batteries for up to 50 hours—there is no excuse for not carrying one. While less useful as a light beacon to be observed from a distance, the dimmer, diffuse light from the LEDs is better for night walking than the brighter, more directed light from incandescent bulbs; your pupils remain sufficiently dilated to see the edge of the trail, and irregularities in the

*HINT: If you decide to descend into the canyon predawn to avoid midday heat, note that when walking downhill in the dark, holding your headlamp at waist level can be useful. Lighting the path at this angle makes shadows that highlight irregularities in the trail.*

trail surface stand out better. For this reason I prefer half-used batteries for night walks.

8. **First-aid kit:** Your first-aid kit will most likely be used to prevent and treat blisters, ease a headache, and dull pain from sore knees. If you sustain a serious injury, it also needs to keep you comfortable and medically stabilized, in case you need to wait to be evacuated.

A basic first-aid kit for a dayhike or short backpacking trip should contain:

- **Sports tape:** This essential first-aid component can be used to prevent or treat blisters, tape anything in place, and provide compression. An ideal anti-blister tape stays in place for many days but isn't too thick; simple, thin, cheap sports tape works well. It stays put and doesn't add bulk to your feet. Many people complain that cheap sports tape rubs off very easily, especially if you have sweaty feet, and recommend using duct tape, but duct tape makes a permanent sticky mess of socks. Another thicker, very sticky tape you might try is Leukoplast (available only in Europe, Australia, and New Zealand, but adored by hikers from those regions).

- **Anti-inflammatory pain medication:** To relieve mild pain and swelling following an injury, ibuprofen, aspirin, and naproxen are all available over the counter. Acetaminophen is not an anti-inflammatory drug, but it is a very effective painkiller. Of these, ibuprofen and acetaminophen are easier on your stomach. If you take any of these, make sure you are well hydrated (to avoid kidney damage) and follow the indications on the product or your physician's advice.

- **Moleskin, blister bandages, or pads:** Examples of blister bandages include Spenco 2nd Skin Blister Pads and Band-Aid Blister Block Cushions. Blister pads are expensive but highly recommended by people with persistent blister problems; these gel pads keep out dirt and germs, while providing cushioning, so your blister won't bother you for the rest of your hike.

- **Elastic bandage:** You may be able to make slow progress down the trail with a strained or sprained ankle or knee wrapped in an elastic bandage. You can also use sports tape for this purpose. Should you be bitten by a rattlesnake, it can also be used as a compression bandage on a limb.

- **Sterile gauze or adhesive pads:** Gauze pads are handy to halt bleeding of a wound. There are many inexpensive brands of adhesive pads to cover wounds. The more expensive

Tegaderm adhesive pads are permeable to water, vapor, and oxygen, but they provide a barrier to microorganisms, making them ideal if you can't reach a doctor for a few hours.

- **Bandages:** Carry a variety of sizes, including butterfly closures. Band-Aids are great for any small cuts, while Steri-Strips can effectively close a larger wound to reduce bleeding.
- **Antibiotic ointment:** Apply antibiotic ointment (triple-action formulas are best) to a wound before dressing it.
- **Antiseptic wipes:** Use wipes to clean a wound before applying dressing.
- **Antihistamine:** Carry an over-the-counter antihistamine in case you have an allergic reaction or allergies. If you are severely allergic to something, you may need to carry something prescription strength, like an EpiPen.
- **Whistle and mirror:** Blow a whistle or use a mirror to signal to attract attention to yourself if you are alone when injured.
- **Tweezers:** Use these to remove splinters.
- **Safety pin:** These are useful for fashioning clothing into slings or large bandages. Large, sturdy ones are handy for small repairs, from broken zippers to backpack straps. Zip ties also work well for fixing broken backpacks.
- **Sterile, nonlatex gloves:** Wear these if you are treating an open wound on another person.
- **Small first-aid book:** Pamphlet-sized books are available at most outdoor stores. It is best to know basic first aid and to be familiar with your book's coverage, only relying on your book to provide details and trigger your memory.
- **Other items** you may choose to carry in your first-aid kit include: a wire splint, chemical hand-warmer packets, prescription pain medication, an anti-diarrhea drug (such as loperamide), and a knee brace.

9. **Fire starter and matches:** You should always carry these. In the Grand Canyon, other than for lighting a camp stove, they should be used only in an emergency, and then only to create a small smoke signal to help rescuers pinpoint your location. Burn only your fire starter and light it in the middle of the trail-the National Park Service prohibits fires below the canyon rim to protect vegetation and avoid a wildfire, a very real danger.

10. **Knife:** A small pocketknife, especially one with a pair of scissors, is important for cutting first-aid supplies—and probably for preparing your lunch.

## DAYHIKE GEAR LIST

In addition to the 10 essentials, dayhikers should carry the following:

- **Daypack:** Any small backpack will work. Some daypacks covered with gadgets and many small pockets can weigh 4 pounds or more, but they aren't necessary for this hike. Pick a simple one. Some people prefer a hip pack, but make sure you bring one that can accommodate a gallon of water.
- **Space blanket:** A space blanket is almost as important as the 10 essentials. One costs less than $5, weighs about 3 ounces, and can help you retain body heat. Remember that even during summer the temperature on the upper trail sections will drop into the low 40s most nights. Using a space blanket will reduce the possibility of hypothermia if you spend an unplanned night on the trail. Keep in mind that any trauma injury can lead to a reduced ability to regulate body temperature.
- **Spray bottle:** A spray bottle is an excellent way to cool yourself. Spray some water on your face or the back of your neck and enjoy some relief.

Optional items include:

- **Trekking poles:** Hikers increasingly carry trekking poles. Their many advantages include taking weight off your knees and toes, transferring some of the "work" to your arms, and providing extra balance, thereby minimizing your risk of falling.
- **Camera:** A camera is hardly optional for most people descending into the Grand Canyon, but it's not required for your safety.
- **Water-treatment method:** Most hikers will opt not to carry this, as treated water is available along the Bright Angel Trail (no water is available on the South Kaibab Trail). However, options are described on page 69.

## OVERNIGHT GEAR LIST

In addition to the 10 essentials and the aforementioned dayhiking gear, backpackers should carry the following:

- **Overnight backpack:** Either an internal or external frame backpack works well.

- **Additional clothes:** During the summer months you shouldn't need more than a lightweight waterproof jacket (if rain is possible), and a thermal top. For excursions in late fall and spring, add a fleece hat, fleece jacket, and thermal bottoms to your pack, especially if you are spending a night at the Indian Garden Campground. In winter, when low temperatures at the bottom of the canyon hover just above freezing bring a down vest, wind or rain pants, and light-weight gloves.

- **Sleeping bag or liner:** In summer, you are likely to use at most a liner (silk or cotton) at the Bright Angel Campground, while most people will wish to have a lightweight (rated to 30 degrees or higher) sleeping bag at the Indian Garden Campground. For spring and fall a 20-degree sleeping bag is a good alternative, but check the weather forecast, as extreme temperatures (in both directions) regularly occur during these months. And, for midwinter conditions, a zero-degree sleeping bag is desirable at all locations.

- **Ground pad:** Bring either a closed-cell foam pad or an inflat-able mattress. To save weight, I carry a short pad and place clothes and my empty backpack under my feet.

- **Tent:** During the warm months a tent serves two purposes: The fly protects you from thundershowers and the tent body protects you from scorpions (see page 68 for more details). If you will be out for only a few nights and the forecast is for clear skies, you can comfortably omit the rainfly from your pack. Many hikers are willing to risk a painful scorpion sting and choose to sleep on a tarp. The true Grand Canyon veterans are identified as those sleeping on the picnic tables—but there is only one per campsite, so claim it ahead of your compan-ions. During the cooler months a tent is desirable for warmth. In winter, if you are expecting a strong storm, a four-season tent (without mesh walls) is the better choice.

*HINT: If you plan to rent gear, the Inner Canyon Backpacker's Shop inside the Canyon Village Marketplace (the general store at Market Plaza) rents and sells most of the equipment you will need, including tents, sleeping bags, ground pads, backpacks, stoves, and trekking poles. Renting here saves you from carrying every-thing on a plane and reduces your rental days. Call 928-638-2262 for more information.*

# PACKING CHECKLIST

| | Dayhike | Overnight | Optional | Season |
|---|---|---|---|---|
| Daypack | ● | | | ALL YEAR |
| Overnight backpack | | ● | | ALL YEAR |
| **Route-Finding** | | | | |
| Map | ● | ● | | ALL YEAR |
| GPS unit | ● | ● | ● | ALL YEAR |
| Compass | ● | ● | | ALL YEAR |
| **Sun Protection** | | | | |
| Sunglasses | ● | ● | | ALL YEAR |
| Sunscreen (SPF 30+) | ● | ● | | ALL YEAR |
| Lip balm (SPF 15+) | ● | ● | | ALL YEAR |
| Sunhat with ear protection | ● | ● | | ALL YEAR |
| **Food & Water** | | | | |
| Food | ● | ● | | ALL YEAR |
| Water bottles or hydration system | ● | ● | | ALL YEAR |
| **Clothes** | | | | |
| Shoes | ● | ● | | ALL YEAR |
| Fleece or wool hat | ● | ● | | SP, F, W |
| Thermal bottoms | ● | ● | | SP, F, W |
| Thermal top | ● | ● | | ALL YEAR |
| Fleece top | ● | ● | | SP, F, W |
| Rain & wind jacket | ● | ● | | ALL YEAR |
| Rain & wind pants | ● | ● | | W |
| Socks (plus extra pair) | ● | ● | | ALL YEAR |
| Shirt | ● | ● | | ALL YEAR |
| Shorts or pants | ● | ● | | ALL YEAR |
| Gaiters | ● | ● | ● | ALL YEAR |
| Gloves | ● | ● | | W |
| Down vest or jacket | ● | ● | | W |

| | Dayhike | Overnight | Optional | Season |
|---|:---:|:---:|:---:|:---:|
| **First-Aid Kit** | | | | |
| ☐ Sports tape | ● | ● | | ALL YEAR |
| ☐ Pain medication | ● | ● | | ALL YEAR |
| ☐ Moleskin or blister bandages | ● | ● | | ALL YEAR |
| ☐ Elastic bandage | ● | ● | | ALL YEAR |
| ☐ Sterile gauze & adhesive pads | ● | ● | | ALL YEAR |
| ☐ Miscellaneous bandages | ● | ● | | ALL YEAR |
| ☐ Antibiotic ointment | ● | ● | | ALL YEAR |
| ☐ Antiseptic wipes | ● | ● | | ALL YEAR |
| ☐ Antihistamine | ● | ● | | ALL YEAR |
| ☐ Whistle & mirror | ● | ● | | ALL YEAR |
| ☐ Tweezers | ● | ● | | ALL YEAR |
| ☐ Safety pin | ● | ● | | ALL YEAR |
| ☐ Sterile gloves | ● | ● | | ALL YEAR |
| ☐ First-aid book | ● | ● | | ALL YEAR |
| **Miscellaneous** | | | | |
| ☐ Headlamp | ● | ● | | ALL YEAR |
| ☐ Fire starter | ● | ● | | ALL YEAR |
| ☐ Matches | ● | ● | | ALL YEAR |
| ☐ Knife | ● | ● | | ALL YEAR |
| ☐ Space blanket | ● | ● | | ALL YEAR |
| ☐ Spray bottle | ● | ● | | SU |
| ☐ Trekking poles | ● | ● | ● | ALL YEAR |
| ☐ Camera | ● | ● | ● | ALL YEAR |
| ☐ Water treatment | ● | ● | ● | ALL YEAR |
| ☐ Tent | | ● | | ALL YEAR |
| ☐ Sleeping bag and/or liner | | ● | | ALL YEAR |
| ☐ Ground pad | | ● | | ALL YEAR |
| ☐ Stove | | ● | | ALL YEAR |
| ☐ Stove fuel | | ● | | ALL YEAR |
| ☐ Cooking pot | | ● | | ALL YEAR |
| ☐ Eating utensil | | ● | | ALL YEAR |
| ☐ Eating vessel | | ● | | ALL YEAR |
| ☐ Toiletry kit | | ● | | ALL YEAR |

- **Stove and fuel:** Stoves with fuel canisters or white gas stoves are good choices. Since campfires are prohibited, all food must be cooked on a stove.
- **Pot:** Any lightweight camping pot works well. A single 2-liter pot works well for up to three people, while larger groups might choose to carry a second pot.
- **Eating utensils and eating container:** Lightweight Lexan cutlery is available at outdoor stores, and a small lightweight plastic bowl is ideal as an eating container.
- **A simple toiletry kit:** Bring a toothbrush and toothpaste, personal medications, extra toilet paper, and tampons or sanitary pads (if applicable). Keep it simple, since toiletry bags can easily become heavy.

# Getting to Grand Canyon Village

The Grand Canyon is located in northern Arizona. The extensive national park runs 277 river miles, from Lees Ferry a little downstream of Lake Powell, near the Utah state border, to Lake Mead at the Nevada border. Most visitors, however, are restricted to a much smaller piece of the landscape by the limited road access. In fact, nearly all visitors gaze at the canyon from Grand Canyon Village on the South Rim, from where the two trails described in this book depart. Many web searches for Grand Canyon information will point you to Tusayan, a community that is a collection of hotels, restaurants, and other tourism-related industries 2 miles south of the national park boundary—a 10-minute drive from the South Rim.

## BY CAR

**Approaching from the south or east and passing through Flagstaff, Arizona:** If you are approaching the Grand Canyon from southern Arizona (e.g., **Phoenix** or **Tucson**), take US 17 north to Flagstaff. Flagstaff is 140 miles north of Phoenix and 260 miles north of Tucson. If you approach from the east (e.g., **Albuquerque,** New Mexico), take Interstate 40 to Flagstaff. Flagstaff is 320 miles west of Albuquerque.

In Flagstaff, turn onto US 180 north toward the Grand Canyon. Follow this small road 42 miles northwest to the small town of

Valle. Turn right onto AZ 64 north and follow it 27 miles to Grand Canyon Village, passing through Tusayan en route.

**Approaching from the west and passing through Williams, Arizona:** If you are approaching from the west (e.g., **Las Vegas** or **Los Angeles**), you will reach the town of Williams (on US 40), and then head north to the Grand Canyon.

From Las Vegas, head toward the intersection of Interstate 215 and Interstate 515 (also posted as US 93 and NV 95) in southeastern Las Vegas. (From the airport you will take I-215 10 miles east to this location.) Continue for 90 miles, crossing into Arizona at Lake Mead and then reaching Interstate 40 in Kingman, Arizona. Continue east on I-40 for 112 miles to Williams, Arizona.

From Los Angeles, head toward I-15 in northeastern Los Angeles, near San Bernardino. (From the Los Angeles International Airport, turn onto Interstate 105 east, following it for 17 miles to Interstate 605. Turn onto I-605 north and follow it 12 miles to Interstate 10. Turn onto I-10 north and follow it for 27 miles to I-15.) From the intersection of I-10 and I-15, head north on I-15 for 73 miles to the intersection with Interstate 40 in Barstow, California. Continue east on I-40 for 315 miles to Williams, Arizona.

In Williams, take exit 165 onto AZ 64. Follow it north 58 miles to Grand Canyon Village, passing Valle and Tusayan en route.

**Approaching from the north and passing through Cameron, Arizona:** From locations to the north including **Zion National Park** (St. George, Utah) and **Arches National Park** (near Moab, Utah), you will enter the Grand Canyon by driving south on US 89 to Cameron, Arizona. In Cameron, turn right onto AZ 64 and head west along the South Rim of the Grand Canyon for 56 miles to Grand Canyon Village. (This road is also called the Desert View Drive.) As there are many different approaches to US 89 at Cameron, consult a map for the best approach from your previous location.

## BY AIR

**Flagstaff:** US Airways Express and Horizon/Alaska Airlines have flights to Flagstaff, approximately one hour southeast of Grand Canyon Village. Once in Flagstaff, you can rent a car or take one of the shuttle services (described below).

**Las Vegas and Phoenix:** Las Vegas and Phoenix have the closest airports serviced by all major airlines.

**Tusayan:** If you do not need to have a car once you arrive in the Grand Canyon, flying into the Grand Canyon Airport in Tusayan is a good choice. Four small airlines currently provide service to this small airport, located 10 minutes south of the entrance to Grand Canyon National Park. They depart from destinations including Las Vegas, Nevada, and Long Beach, California. See www.grand-canyonairport.net for current contact information. In summer, the national park provides a free shuttle service from Tusayan into the park. In addition, Xanterra South Rim provides a taxi service (see opposite page).

## BY TRAIN

The Grand Canyon Railway travels daily between Williams, Arizona, and the South Rim of the Grand Canyon, departing Williams mid-morning and returning in the evening. The 84-mile journey takes two hours and fifteen minutes each direction. As the schedule varies by season, visit www.thetrain.com for details and pack-aged rates that include hotel stays in Williams or Grand Canyon Village. Since your starting point is unlikely to be Williams, visit the Amtrak website (www.amtrak.com) for information about con-nections. (Williams lies on the Amtrak route *Southwest Chief* that travels from Los Angeles to Flagstaff to Albuquerque and eastward to Chicago.)

## SHUTTLE, BUS, AND TAXI SERVICES

**Open Road Tours** (928-226-8060 or 877-226-8060) offers morning and afternoon bus service from Flagstaff to Williams and then on to Grand Canyon Village. Buses run between Phoenix and Flagstaff five times a day. Visit www.openroadtours.com for additional information.

**Arizona Shuttle** (928-266-8060 or 877-226-8060) offers three trips daily from Flagstaff direct to Grand Canyon Village. Buses run between Phoenix and Flagstaff seven times a day. Visit www.arizo-nashuttle.com for additional information.

**Greyhound Bus Lines** (800-231-2222 or 928-774-4573 for the Flagstaff office) has stops in Flagstaff and Williams, and both shuttle services listed above stop at the Greyhound depot in Flagstaff. Visit www.greyhound.com for additional information.

**Xanterra South Rim** (928-638-2822), the South Rim concessionaire, offers a taxi service to Tusayan, including the Grand Canyon Airport. (However, from mid-May to mid-September, the national park provides a free shuttle line, the Purple Line.)

Visit www.nps.gov/grca/planyourvisit/publictransportation.htm for additional information on public transportation.

# Getting Around Grand Canyon Village

Several free shuttle lines operate out of Grand Canyon Village, allowing you to travel around the area without a car. Indeed, you must leave your car at the Backcountry Information Center when you embark on your walk and either walk (for the Bright Angel Trail) or take a shuttle (for the South Kaibab Trail) to the trailhead. See centerfold of *The South Rim Guide*, the newspaper you receive when you enter the park for a map of shuttle routes.

If you do have a car with you, you will likely decide to take it to your campsite or hotel and park it at the Backcountry Information Center just before beginning your walk. However, if you have days before or after your hike to tour the South Rim, park it for the day at the Backcountry Information Center and take the shuttles; the frustration of trying to find one of the limited number of parking spots is not worth the convenience of having a car.

The Blue Line, or Village Route, circles Grand Canyon Village itself, including the Backcountry Information Center, campgrounds (see below), and Yavapai Point with stops at Market Plaza, Mather Campground, and the various lodges. If you are descending the Bright Angel Trail, leave your car at the Backcountry Information Center and either walk a half mile or take the Blue Line to the start of the hike. (Walking is faster in this case.)

The Green Line, or Kaibab Trail Route, is the only way to reach the South Kaibab Trailhead, as cars are not permitted there from March to November. It departs from the Canyon View Information Plaza (also called the Grand Canyon Visitor Center), the eastern extent of the Blue Line. You should park at the Backcounty Information Center and take the Blue Line to this location. (Note that the roads accessing the Canyon View Information Plaza and a large parking lot at this location are currently under construction. The shuttles used to stop at Mather Point, a five-minute walk north of the Information Plaza.)

In addition there is the early morning Hiker's Express Shuttle from the Bright Angel Lodge and Backcountry Information Center to the South Kaibab Trailhead, the most efficient option for reaching that trailhead. Departure times, which change monthly to match the changing sunrise and temperature conditions, are listed below.

| Month | Departure Times |
|---|---|
| December, January, and February | 8 and 9 A.M. |
| March and November | 7, 8, and 9 A.M. |
| April and October | 6, 7, and 8 A.M. |
| May and September | 5, 6, and 7 A.M. |
| June, July, and August | 4, 5, and 6 A.M. |

# Grand Canyon Village and Tusayan Services

## LODGING AND CAMPING OPTIONS

There are a multitude of lodging options in the vicinity of the South Rim of the Grand Canyon. Those inside the national park offer the advantage that on the day of your departure you can just hop on a shuttle bus or walk down a trail, but there are far more rooms in Tusayan and beyond. Tusayan has several large hotels, but rooms tend to be pricey. Williams and Flagstaff, an hour from the South Rim, offer considerably cheaper accommodation. If you plan to drive into the park the morning you begin your walk, these can be good alternatives. Look through their chamber of commerce websites to find local lodging choices: www.williamschamber.com and www.flagstaffchamber.com.

### Grand Canyon Village Hotels

There are six lodges and hotels in Grand Canyon Village, all run by Xanterra Parks & Resorts, the concessionaire at the South Rim. For reservations call 888-297-2757 (in advance) or 928-638-2631 (same day). In order of cost, they are: Bright Angel (and cabins), Maswik,

Yavapai, Kachina, and Thunderbird lodges, and El Tovar Hotel. See www.grandcanyonlodges.com for additional information.

### Tusayan Hotels and Motels

There are five large hotels in Tusayan. Since the U.S. Postal Service name for Tusayan is "Grand Canyon," they all have "Grand Canyon, AZ" addresses. The Tusayan chamber of commerce website (www. grandcanyonchamber.com) includes lodging options outside Tusayan—if you look at these listings, make sure your reservation is for a Tusayan (Grand Canyon) location.

**Best Western Grand Canyon Squire Inn**
928-638-2681 or 800-622-6966
www.grandcanyonsquire.com

**Grand Canyon Plaza Resort**
928-638-2673 or 800-995-2521
www.grandcanyonplaza.com

**The Grand Hotel**
928-638-3333 or 888-634-7263
www.grandcanyongrandhotel.com

**Holiday Inn Express**
928-638-3000
www.gcanyon.com

**Red Feather Lodge**
928-638-2414 or 866-561-2425
www.redfeatherlodge.com

### RV Facilities

**Grand Canyon National Park:**

**Trailer Village**
Located between Mather Campground and the Marketplace, Trailer Village is run by the concessionaire, Xanterra Parks & Resorts. For reservations call 888-297-2757 (in advance) or 928-638-2631 (same day). The cost is $32 for two adults and $2 for each additional adult.

**Tusayan:**

### Camper Village

Located near the north end of Tusayan, this private campground has 294 sites. Tents are welcome, although it is targeted to RVs. There are showers, laundry, and a small on-site store. Reservations can be made online at www.grandcanyoncampervillage.com or by calling 928-638-2887 or 800-638-2887. The cost is $20 for tents and $30–43 for RVs depending on hookups at the site (water, sewer, and electricity).

## *Camping*

### Grand Canyon National Park:

### Mather Campground

Located near Market Plaza, this lovely campground has 327 sites. Reservations are recommended and can be made at www.recreation.gov or by calling 877-444-6777. The cost is $18 for single sites ($15 in winter). Amenities include water, flush toilets (and heated bathrooms with power outlets), free dump station, showers, and laundry (both at an additional cost). RV hook-ups are not available.

### Desert View Campground

Located 25 miles (a 45-minute drive) east of Grand Canyon Village near the Desert View vista and the Watchtower, this summer-only campground has 50 first-come, first-served sites. They cost $12 per night, and amenities include water and flush toilets, but RV hook-ups are not available.

### Kaibab National Forest:

### Ten-X Campground

Located 4.3 miles south of the national park entrance station (2 miles south of Tusayan), this campground has 70 first-come, first-served sites and two group campsites that can be reserved. The cost is $10 for single sites per night, and amenities include water and pit toilets (there aren't RV hook-ups). See www.fs.fed.us/r3/kai/recreation/campgrounds/TenX.shtml for additional information.

Dispersed camping (camping in unimproved sites, i.e., by the side of a dirt road) is allowed in Kaibab National Forest, as long as you are a quarter mile from water. The ranger station just north of Tusayan can provide a map with suggested locations.

## RESTAURANTS

Several places inside Grand Canyon National Park serve food. These restaurants' seasonal hours are given in *The Guide*, the newspaper handed out at the park entrance. At Market Plaza, check out Canyon Café (in Yavapai Lodge) or Delicatessen (in the General Store). In Grand Canyon Village, you can choose from Maswik Cafeteria (in Maswik Lodge, across the train tracks from the Backcountry Office), Bright Angel Restaurant (in Bright Angel Lodge), The Arizona Room (also in Bright Angel Lodge), and El Tovar Dining Room (in El Tovar Hotel and requires reservations for dinner).

Tusayan has many additional choices. If you are camping, the General Store at Market Plaza has a very good selection of food.

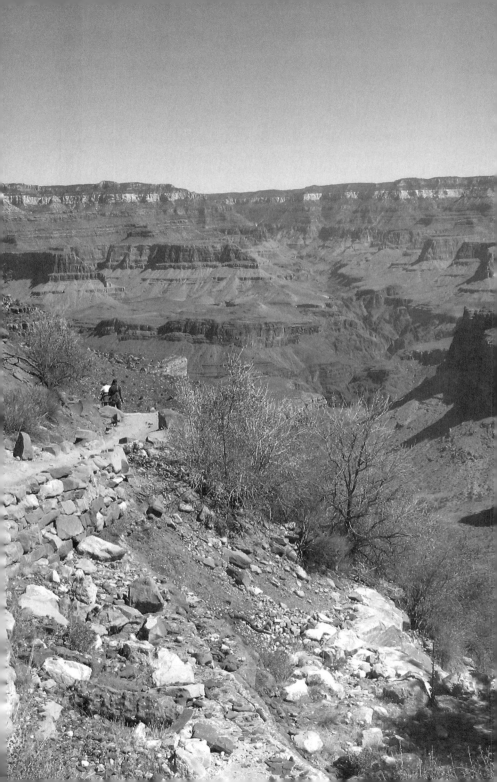

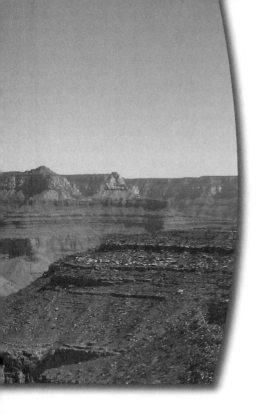

# 4

# Hiking the Grand Canyon

These detailed descriptions of the South Kaibab and Bright Angel trails, include sketch maps, shaded relief maps based on digital elevation models, and elevation profiles. Of the four suggestions for side trips, three are from the Bright Angel Campground and one is from the Indian Garden Campground. The descriptions of terrain have a healthy dose of geology and biology. If you want additional information, refer to the natural history section of this book (see page 15) and consider reading some of the additional geology references listed in the bibliography (see page 164).

## Suggested Schedules

Much as I—and the park service—dissuade you from attempting a dayhike, both dayhiking and backpacking itineraries are covered. *For both dayhikes and overnight trips, if it is hot, start at dawn and take breaks. If it is cold, the days are probably short, so still start early.*

*Opposite and above:* Approaching the 1.5-Mile Resthouse on the Bright Angel Trail

## DAYHIKING

Hikers completing this hike in a day are risking their safety and take in less of the canyon experience than those taking more time. Only people who frequently take long, steep hikes, are familiar with desert hiking conditions, and, if it is hot, are acclimatized to heat (see page 83) should attempt this hike. Don't descend below the Tonto Platform if the high temperature at Phantom Ranch is forecasted to be above 85°F. If you cannot be dissuaded from dayhiking, be smart, and ensure that your schedule allows plenty of time for breaks and that you are carrying the necessary gear (see page 102).

Precisely 9.4 miles of the trail is on descending, flat, or gently ascending terrain (from the South Kaibab Trailhead to where you leave Pipe Creek at the base of Devils Corkscrew) and the remaining 6.7 miles is a steep ascent. Including short breaks, most dayhikers will descend and walk on even ground at a rate of about 2 miles an hour, requiring about 5 hours to reach the base of Devils Corkscrew. This time includes 10 minutes of breaks per hour, but not longer breaks for lunch or shady siestas. Then comes the ascent.

The rule of thumb for backpackers is that one ascends at a rate of 2 miles per hour plus an extra hour for each thousand feet of elevation gain. Based on this calculation, the 4100-foot climb from the base of Devils Corkscrew to the Bright Angel Trailhead takes nearly 8 hours. Dayhikers carry less weight—although still a hefty amount of water—and may take as little as 4 hours, or possibly more than 8 hours. Your total roundtrip walking time, including short breaks, but excluding lunch breaks, will range from 8 to 14 hours, with many taking around 12 hours. In other words, a very long day.

*HINT: It is especially important for dayhikers to take it easy on the way down—you must have sufficient energy to retrace your steps the same day.*

Even ignoring the likelihood that you will need to hole up due to midday heat, you need to embark on a 12-hour hike very early in the morning. During the winter months there are not 12 hours of daylight, making the walk impractical, since you will need to negotiate the upper, often icy, stretches of trail by headlamp. During the spring and fall, the best times for a dayhike, you should begin no later than sunrise, taking one of the early morning direct hiker shuttles (see page 106). During the summer months, it is very ill advised to dayhike, since you will be spending most of your walk hiking in temperatures surpassing 80°F—and without shade. For approximate temperatures for a mid-June hike, see figure on page 77.

## BACKPACKING

Backpackers who complete the 16.1-mile loop over 2 days, with a night at Bright Angel Campground, will on the first day descend 6.8 miles from the South Kaibab Trailhead to the campground. The second day will include 2.6 miles of flat to gently ascending terrain, from the Bright Angel Campground to where they leave Pipe Creek to ascend the Devils Corkscrew, and 6.7 miles of a steep climb to the Bright Angel Trailhead, a total elevation gain of 4600 feet. Backpackers who split the ascent with a night at Indian Garden will, on their first day, complete the 2.6 miles of gentle terrain and the first 2 miles of the climb. On their second day they will climb another 4.7 miles and 3000 feet of elevation.

### *The Descent*

If you are backpacking, the 6.8-mile descent of the South Kaibab Trail is not long in hours. A fast hiker will descend in as little as 3 hours while someone seeking a leisurely pace will stretch the

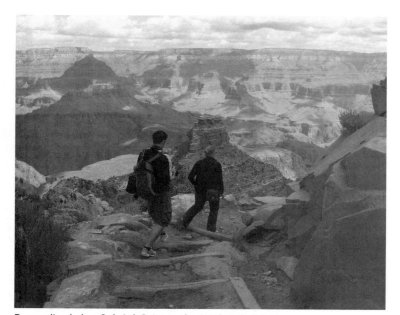

Descending below Ooh Aah Point on the South Kaibab Trail

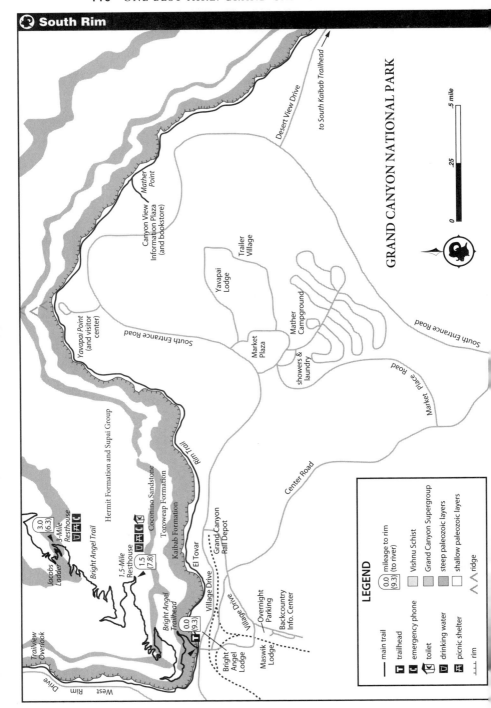

GRAND CANYON NATIONAL PARK

to South Kaibab Trailhead

Desert View Drive

Mather Point

Canyon View Information Plaza (and bookstore)

Trailer Village

Yavapai Lodge

Yavapai Point (and visitor center)

Mather Campground

South Entrance Road

Market Plaza

showers & laundry

South Entrance Road

Market Place Road

Hermit Formation and Supai Group

Coconino Sandstone

Toroweap Formation

Kaibab Formation

Rim Trail

Center Road

3.0
(6.3)

3-Mile Resthouse

Jacobs Ladder

Bright Angel Trail

1.5-Mile Resthouse

1.5
7.8

El Tovar

Grand Canyon Rail Depot

Village Drive

Trailview Overlook

West Rim Drive

Bright Angel Trailhead

0.0
(9.3)

Village Drive

Overnight Parking

Backcountry Info. Center

Bright Angel Lodge

Maswik Lodge

0    .25    .5 mile

**LEGEND**

— main trail

▬ trailhead

☎ emergency phone

🚻 toilet

💧 drinking water

⛱ picnic shelter

⌄⌄ rim

0.0  mileage to rim
(9.3) (to river)

Vishnu Schist

Grand Canyon Supergroup

steep paleozoic layers

shallow paleozoic layers

∧∧ ridge

descent over 6 hours. These estimates include 10 minutes of breaks each hour. Many people will also take a long lunch break, increasing their total descent time. These times are, on average, longer than the backpacker's rule of thumb that it takes an hour to backpack 2 miles on level or descending terrain. Although well maintained and graded, this trail is still tough walking; it has numerous steps, sections with potholes, and a persistent grade.

The descent will not require all daylight hours, but it is still essential that you begin early. From May through September the Inner Gorge temperatures are sufficiently hot that you will not particularly enjoy (or worse) the walk below Skeleton Point after midmorning and will likely feel exhausted when you reach the bottom. Begin your hike around sunrise to best appreciate your surroundings and minimize the likelihood of heat-related injuries. Conveniently, the Hiker's Express Shuttles (see page 107) are timed to keep you on this schedule. During the cooler months mornings are nippy at the South Rim, and you can hike during much of the day; you will have sufficient time if you begin by midmorning.

### The Ascent

As with the descent, the number of hours required for the hike is limited, not by daylight (except in midwinter), but instead by the number of daylight hours when walking is comfortable. The 9.3 miles of trail from Bright Angel Campground to the Bright Angel Trailhead, including a few shorts "descents" along the River Trail, climbs nearly 4600 feet.

The first 2.6 miles, to where you leave Pipe Creek, are flat to gently ascending, followed by 6.7 notably steep miles. The standard backpacker's estimate that one ascends at a rate of 2 miles per hour plus an extra hour for each thousand feet of elevation gain is accurate for this first stretch of trail—it takes approximately 2 hours to hike the 2.6 miles and climb 555 feet to the base of Devils Corkscrew in the cool of the morning.

Completing the 6.7-mile ascent varies much more by person and the weather. It takes between 5 and 10 hours, with 7 hiking hours being a standard estimate for a not too hot day. The backpacker's rule of thumb suggests this climb takes a little less than 6½ hours, a slight underestimate, since backpackers are usually not faced with such a long uphill climb. Most people will begin the climb at a faster clip than the estimate, but will slow as the climb continues and the legs, lungs, and sweat glands begin to complain and the day grows ever hotter. The climb from the Devils Corkscrew to Indian Garden requires about 2 hours and the upper section of the walk an additional 5 hours on average (ranging from 3 to 7 hours, depending on your pace).

During hot weather it is essential to begin your walk early, whether you are heading to Indian Garden or all the way to the rim. The Inner Gorge will reach 80°F within a few hours of sunrise—or sooner—and you want to have made use of your early morning hours. Most people heed this advice, for the Bright Angel Campground is awake by an hour before sunrise, with many campsites empty by the time headlamps can be turned off. In winter, those headed for Indian Garden can have a leisurely morning, since they have only 4.5 miles to go. However if you plan to exit in a single day, leave by 8 A.M. since daylight is limited.

As you climb, remember the ascent is not a race against the mules— who take a little less than 2½ hours from Indian Garden to the rim. Don't be hard on yourself if your pace slows on the upper stretches of the trail. Take your time, take 10 minutes of breaks each hour (included in these estimates), take one or more long lunch breaks (not included in these estimates), enjoy the surroundings, seek shady hideouts, and simply plan to reach the canyon rim in the late afternoon or evening.

## REMINDERS FOR YOUR WALK

- Leave the top of the South Kaibab Trail carrying 3 liters of water.
- Leave the Colorado River carrying 3 liters of water.
- From Indian Garden to the top of the Bright Angel Trail, top off your water at each faucet (Indian Garden and the two resthouses), such that you begin each section of trail with 2 liters.
- Take a 10-minute break each hour, even on the way down.
- If you are uncomfortably hot, find some shade if possible, drink some water, and take a long break.

# South Kaibab Trail

The South Kaibab Trail is usually selected as the descent route, as it is the steeper trail and nearly lacking in shade—but its expansive vistas should not be missed.

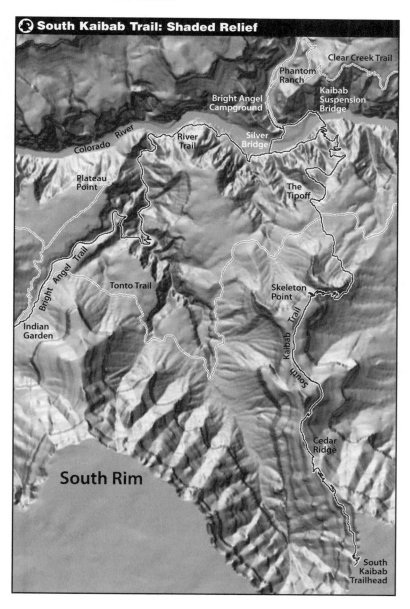

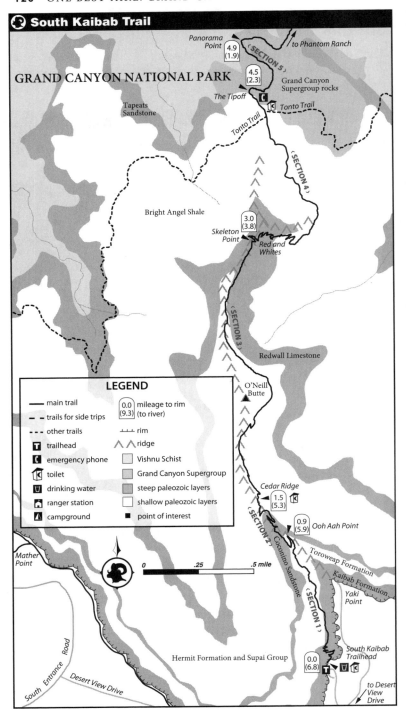

# South Kaibab Trail

GRAND CANYON NATIONAL PARK

Panorama Point ▲ 4.9 (1.9)  ⟨SECTION 5⟩  to Phantom Ranch

4.5 (2.3)  Grand Canyon Supergroup rocks

Tapeats Sandstone

The Tipoff  🅲  Tonto Trail

Tonto Trail

⟨SECTION 4⟩

Bright Angel Shale

3.0 (3.8)

Skeleton Point ▲  Red and Whites

⟨SECTION 3⟩

Redwall Limestone

O'Neill Butte ▲

## LEGEND

— main trail
- - trails for side trips
- - - other trails
🅣 trailhead
🅲 emergency phone
🚻 toilet
🚰 drinking water
🏠 ranger station
🅰 campground

(0.0) mileage to rim
(9.3) (to river)
⊥⊥⊥ rim
∧∧ ridge
▢ Vishnu Schist
▢ Grand Canyon Supergroup
▢ steep paleozoic layers
▢ shallow paleozoic layers
■ point of interest

Cedar Ridge ▲ 1.5 (5.3) 🚻

0.9 (5.9) Ooh Aah Point

Toroweap Formation

⟨SECTION 2⟩

Coconino Sandstone

Kaibab Formation

⟨SECTION 1⟩

Yaki Point

Mather Point

0 .25 .5 mile

Hermit Formation and Supai Group

0.0 (6.8)  South Kaibab Trailhead  🅣 🚰 🚻

South Entrance Road

Desert View Drive

to Desert View Drive

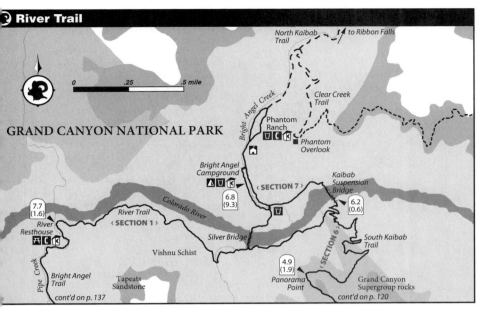

**Note:** The geologic boundaries shown on these trail maps are derived from the geologic map published by the U.S. Geological Survey. Because of the map's large scale, the boundaries shown may not precisely match what you see along the trail.

## SECTION 1

### Canyon Rim to Ooh Aah Point
**Distance** . . . . . . . . . . . . . . 0.9 mile

During most of the year, the spur road to the trailhead and adjacent Yaki Point is closed to private vehicles, and you will take the shuttle to the starting point. At the trailhead make sure you have sufficient water; if you haven't already done so, fill up at the tap near the corral as you walk to the canyon rim. Read and consider the posted warnings and prepare to begin your descent. You first descend a series of tight switchbacks, known as the Chimney, through the Kaibab Limestone, a steep layer that forms an impenetrable

*HINT: While descending most hikers move too quickly to notice the surrounding rock. If you wish to stare at the rock beds, look at the maps above, opposite, and on page 137 to note where the trail crosses each rock type. The South Kaibab and Bright Angel chapters from Abbott and Cook's* Hiking the Grand Canyon's Geology *are excellent trail references.*

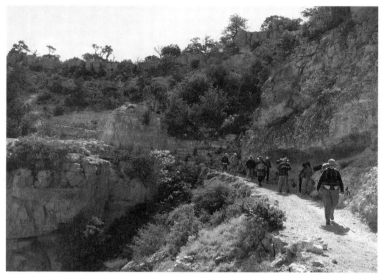

Descending through the Chimney, the first switchbacks on the South Kaibab Trail

wall along much of the rim. Fossil remnants of sponges and shells are readily visible in this light-colored rock.

As you begin a northward traverse below and to the west of the Yaki Point road, you cross into the Toroweap Formation, a stratum composed of interlayered limestone, siltstone, and sandstone. It also includes salt and gypsum deposits, two minerals that formed as water evaporated in an ancient desert environment. The Toroweap's sediments erode to form the sparsely treed sloping bench the trail follows.

After 1 mile you cross into the Coconino Sandstone, a steep, imposing layer that usually blocks downward travel in the Grand Canyon. Stop and look at the amphitheater to the southwest (left) and the next promontory to the west, Mather Point. Throughout this region the Coconino Sandstone creates a 350-foot-tall cliff. Only occasionally where there are narrow ridges, such as the one along which this trail was constructed, has this stratum begun to erode. As you continue northward, you will notice long, diagonal stripes within the Coconino Sandstone. This cross-bedding records the orientation of sloping layers of sand in what were once tall sand dunes. The trail continues its northward trajectory, cutting slowly down through the Coconino Sandstone until you reach Ooh Aah Point, where a panorama suddenly opens to the northeast.

## Ooh Aah Point to Cedar Ridge
**Distance** . . . . . . . . . . . . . . 0.6 mile

Below Ooh Aah Point the trail switch-backs down to the bottom of the Coconino Sandstone. Admire the stone-work along this section; sections of the South Kaibab Trail have just been rebuilt and great care has been taken to build a trail that will survive many decades of feet and hooves. You now enter the red-colored Hermit Formation, sandstone interbedded with more readily eroded

*HINT: Even though you are moving downhill and have probably been walking for less than an hour, stop for 10 minutes when you get to Cedar Ridge to take a big drink and eat and snack. Not overdoing it will pay back later.*

siltstone and mudstone that create a gentler slope. Your views across the canyon and along the precipice below the South Rim are exquisite throughout this section. Shortly, you reach Cedar Ridge, a "flat" perch that offers a toilet and rest areas beneath scattered pinyon pines and junipers—there are no cedars, but junipers have shaggy reddish bark reminiscent of them. To the west of the trail at Cedar Ridge, under a small protective case, is a collection of primi-tive fern fossils.

## Cedar Ridge to Skeleton Point
**Distance** . . . . . . . . . . . . . . 1.5 miles

In this part of the Grand Canyon the Hermit and Supai forma-tions generally form a single long slope between the near-vertical Coconino Sandstone and underlying Redwall Formation, broken only by short outcrops of sandstone. However, here they form the long narrow ridge that stretches from Cedar Ridge to Skeleton Point. Although this stretch of landscape is not horrifically steep, note from the elevation profile (see page 151) that the trail's grade is nearly the same as when cutting through the near-vertical rock layers. The difference? Here there are no switchbacks.

Beyond Cedar Ridge you descend briefly on the east side of the ridge and then again intersect the crest at the saddle just south of O'Neill Butte, the last good place to look west and admire the amphitheater that descends from Mather Point to Pipe Creek. You also have an excellent view of the Tonto Platform between the South Kaibab and Bright Angel trails.

Descending again, skirt the east side of steep-sided O'Neill Butte, enjoying views to the northeast, where Zoroaster Temple and Wotans Throne are prominent. You are now sufficiently below and distant from the canyon rim that you begin to feel that you are part of the inner canyon landscape of buttes and side canyons, rather than enjoying it from above. Along this stretch of trail, my eyes keep drifting to the next ridge east, Pattie Butte, staring at the various rock slides and wondering if it is possible to piece together routes through the cliffs.

Beyond O'Neill Butte, the trail follows a narrow stretch of ridgeline, skirts east of a second small knob, and reaches a nearly flat site dotted with abundant century plants, a species of agave. The century plants on the plateau provide an engaging foreground for landscape photos throughout the year. At the far side of the plateau a short spur trail trends left to Skeleton Point, worth a detour for both the panorama and the view straight down to Garden Creek.

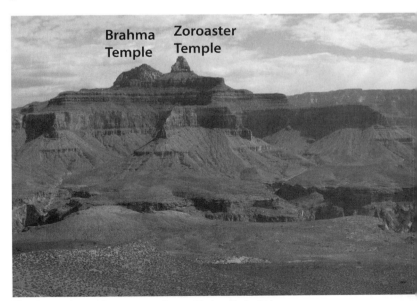

The vista to the northeast as you descend below Cedar Ridge

SECTION
4

# Skeleton Point to The Tipoff
**Distance**............... 1.5 miles

You have now descended more than 2000 feet. But from Skeleton Point, where you can first view the river, you realize your destination is still a long way down. Just beyond Skeleton Point you cross from the Supai Group onto the Redwall Limestone and resume a steep descent rate. After a few steep, exposed switchbacks, you cross a small saddle, look north to a pinnacle of Redwall Limestone, and begin a long set of switchbacks. The Redwall Limestone is another of the layers where descent routes can be difficult to find. East of Skeleton Point this layer has eroded such that the cliffs bands are broken by sections of steep talus that provide a passage, in part because a small fault lies here, breaking up the rock. Juniper logs laid across the trail to prevent erosion create a series of never-ending short steps. Partway down the switchbacks you cross onto the Muav Limestone, a more easily eroded layer, and soon begin a descending traverse around the eastern side of an impressive limestone cliff.

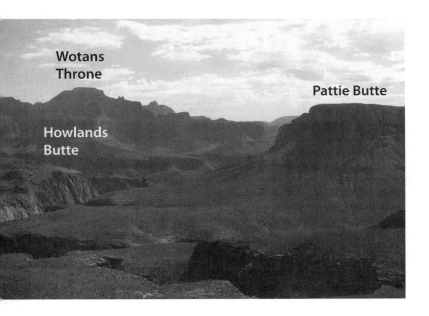

Wotans Throne

Pattie Butte

Howlands Butte

## ROCK DESCRIPTIONS

Below are field descriptions (what the rock looks like) of each of the rock formations you will encounter along the South Kaibab and Bright Angel trails. The geology section (pages 16–27) provides details on the historical environments under which each stratum was deposited and what tectonic conditions led to a given environment.

**Kaibab Formation:** This 350-foot-thick, light-colored limestone layer is not a continuous wall; thin layers of sandstone and siltstone are interbedded within the limestone. This layer has abundant fossils, especially sponges and coral.

**Toroweap Formation:** The Toroweap is also a collection of limestone, sandstone, and siltstone layers. Here, however, the siltstone is dominant, eroding into a lower angle, tree-covered slope. The sandstone and siltstone stand out as steeper beds. The stratum include evaporite deposits (minerals such as gypsum and salt) that are light colored and, at the time of formation, rose above the surrounding sediment, such that they occasionally form small "salt domes" in the rock.

**Coconino Sandstone:** A 350-foot-thick vertical layer of light-colored sandstone in which often-steep cross-bedding is visible, the Coconino forms a barrier to descent along much of the Grand Canyon.

**Hermit Formation:** This stratum is composed of interbedded red siltstone and sandstone. (The red color results from oxidized iron-minerals in the desert-derived sediments that form the rock.) The siltstone layers decompose into a slope, while the sandstone stands out as short, steep beds.

**Supai Group:** This collection of four strata includes the Esplanade Sandstone (uppermost layer) and three slope-forming strata: the Wescogame, Manakacha, and Watahomigi formations. The Esplanade forms a prominent red cliff, which defines the upper walls of the two most prominent buttes along this route: O'Neill Butte and the Battleship (along the Bright Angel Trail). The remaining strata are interbedded limestone, siltstone, and sandstone, which erode into a slope quite similar to that formed on the Hermit Formation: a gradual treed slope interspersed with short, steep sandstone outcrops.

**Redwall Limestone:** The Redwall Limestone forms a 350-foot-thick, steep red cliff. Geologic descriptions indicate it is "light gray" in color, and so it is beneath the surface. Its color derives from reddish pigments in the overlying Hermit and Supai formations that wash down: Where the Redwall Limestone forms the uppermost layer, as is the case in some inner canyon buttes and north of Skeleton Point, it is a lighter color. The stratum erodes, in part, by dissolution of the limestone, such that the Redwall Limestone forms beautiful amphitheaters and contains extensive cave systems.

Along the Bright Angel Trail, a thin lens of material, termed the Surprise Canyon Formation overlies the Redwall Limestone in the vicinity of the 3-Mile Resthouse. Along both trails, lenses of the Temple Butte Limestone exist below the Redwall Limestone. Both strata represent sediment that filled in river channels that had eroded, respectively, in the Redwall Limestone and underlying Muav Limestone.

**Muav Limestone:** The boundary between the Redwall Limestone and the top of the Muav Limestone can be difficult to identify, as they together form a single wall. Lower down, the Muav has a brownish hue, very distinct from the Redwall's color, and forms a more gradual slope interspersed with steep outcrops.

**Bright Angel Shale:** The very easily eroded greenish Bright Angel Shale forms the Tonto Platform. Trace fossils, especially worm tracks, are common in this layer, but as outcrops are infrequent, they are best seen in rocks used to line the South Kaibab Trail. The boundary between the Bright Angel Shale and the Muav Limestone is indistinct, as the two are interbedded where they meet.

**Tapeats Sandstone:** This light-colored sandstone has steep walls with obvious bedding planes. Along both trails, its start is immediately obvious, for it marks the end of the Tonto Platform. This layer is 300 feet thick along the Bright Angel Trail, but quite thin along the South Kaibab Trail due to faulting.

**Unkar Group formations:** From top to bottom the Unkar Group of the Grand Canyon Supergroup is composed of the Cardenas Lava, Dox Formation, Shinumo Quartzite, Hakatai Shale, and Bass Limestone. Only the bottom three of these strata outcrop along the South Kaibab Trail (and none along the Bright Angel Trail). Shinumo Quartzite is a purplish-red silica cemented sandstone. That is, it has not been metamorphosed as the name quartzite indicates, but the particles are cemented together with silica, making it as hard as a quartzite. Only the bottom section is present where it outcrops along the South Kaibab Trail. The Hakatai Shale is a bright orange-and-red layer of fairly easily eroded rock in which fine bedding can sometimes be seen. Ripple marks and mud cracks are visible in places. Varying from rough gray to orange, Bass Limestone contains stromatolites, some of the first primitive life on Earth and the oldest fossils in the Grand Canyon. They appear as wavy layers within the rock.

**Vishnu Schist and Zoroaster Granite:** The Inner Gorge is comprised of a collection of schists and granites dating from plate collisions 1.7 to 1.4 billion years ago. Schist is a metamorphic rock that forms when existing rock is subjected to sufficiently high temperatures and pressures that the individual minerals are flattened. Schists are dark colored, some massive and others layered. The type of rock that was metamorphosed differentiates the various schists. For instance, the Vishnu Schist is layered; these foliations are remnants of the layered sediments that were metamorphosed. In contrast, the Brahma and Rama schists are derived from volcanic rocks and lack layers. Granite is an intrusive igneous rock, a rock that solidified underground from magma. Zoroaster Granite is pink because of its high concentrations of the mineral potassium feldspar.

The landscape becomes even gentler where you cross onto the Bright Angel Shale, the stratum that forms the expansive Tonto Platform. While the Muav Limestone was brownish to grayish in color, the Bright Angel Shale has a greenish hue from the mineral glauconite. Look up while walking down the west-trending stretch of trail; there is a natural arch high up in the Redwall Limestone.

The Tonto Platform is covered with blackbrush, a shrub that predominates across large swaths of undisturbed land at about this elevation throughout the Southwest. It loses its leaves by summer, displaying a thicket of blackish branches. The trail bears nearly due north across the Tonto, crossing the more lightly traveled east and west Tonto trails shortly before reaching some toilets, and a short distance later, an emergency phone. Just as you see the side trail to the phone, you cross into the Tapeats Sandstone, a less-easily eroded layer that forms vertical, beige walls. Here the walls are not tall because the layer has been sliced by the Tipoff Fault, but along the Bright Angel Trail it forms a 300-foot-high wall. You pass through a short distance of Tapeats Narrows as the trail bends to the right. Now the landscape drops off again—you're at the Tipoff.

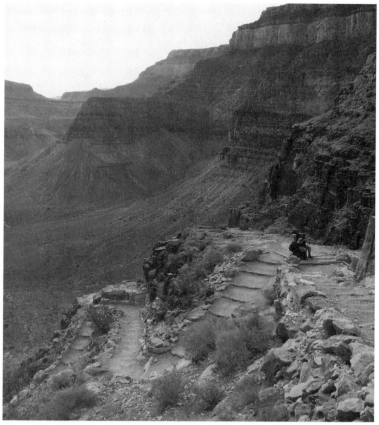

Descending switchbacks below Skeleton Point with a view to the southeast

## SECTION 5

# The Tipoff to Panorama Point

**Distance** . . . . . . . . . . . . . . 0.4 mile

*HINT: Don't rush—you have plenty of time. Stop for rest breaks and to admire the rock layers and plants.*

The stretch of the South Kaibab Trail from the Tipoff to the Kaibab Suspension Bridge predated the 1925 construction of the trail. Known as the Cable Trail, the old (much steeper) trail descended from the Tonto Platform to the Colorado River, where a cable stretched across the river—the only dry route across before the first bridge was constructed in 1921. Prior to the construction of the River Trail in 1936, hikers who wished to cross the Colorado River descended the Bright Angel Trail to the Tonto Trail (just beyond Indian Garden), followed the Tonto Trail to the Tipoff, and the Cable Trail to the Colorado River.

Shortly after you begin a long east-trending switchback, the Tapeats Sandstone ends and you cross onto Shinumo Quartzite, one of the Grand Canyon Supergroup strata. Even before you leave the Tapeats, your eye will likely be drawn to a long northwest-trending stretch of trail a short distance ahead, for the rock, the Hakatai Shale, is a rich burgundy and the layers within the rock are

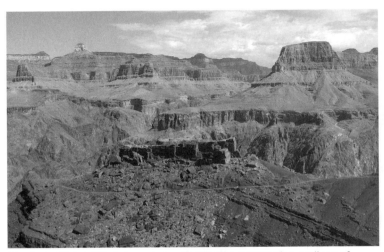

The slanted Hakatai Shale layers below the Tipoff contrast with a small cap of horizontal Tapeats Sandstone.

clearly not parallel to a small steep block of rock above the trail, a cap of Tapeats Sandstone. In fact, unlike all the rock layers from the canyon rim through the Tapeats Sandstone, which are nearly horizontal, the Grand Canyon Supergroup encompasses a much older collection of rocks that were tilted before the deposition of the overlying, newer sediments. The presence of these rocks along South Kaibab Trail is special because in many places in the Grand Canyon the Supergroup strata are missing: After their deposition, they were uplifted and subsequently eroded until nothing remained, such that the Tapeats lies directly atop the basement rocks of the Inner Gorge. Here you are walking through a geologic graben, or grave, where a pair of faults lowered a section of Supergroup strata relative to surrounding rocks. They therefore survived the erosion to which the areas to the east and west were subjected.

Along the northward stretch with the slanting maroon layers, you are walking on Hakatai Shale, which formed in a shallow water environments. This brings you to Panorama Point, a vista just a minute's walk beyond the trail that boasts a superb view down to the Kaibab Bridge and the mouth of Bright Angel Creek.

## SECTION 6  Panorama Point to Kaibab Suspension Bridge
Distance. . . . . . . . . . . . . . 1.1 miles

Beyond Panorama Point, the trail makes a tight turn, and continues for another stretch through the Grand Canyon Supergroup strata. You cross the Hakatai Shale and briefly cross into the rough-textured Bass Limestone before reaching the first outcrops of basement rocks. Because of faulting you cross back into Bass Limestone again, at a location where wavy bedding that indicates the presence of stromatolites, or primitive bacterial mats, is obvious. As you begin descending a set of tighter switchbacks you cross into the basement rocks again, the dark gray Vishnu Schist and pinkish Zoroaster Granite, which together form the steep walls of the Inner Gorge. The trail winds down the final 800 feet to the Kaibab Bridge, mostly staying near a small ridgeline where the rock walls are partially eroded, allowing passage.

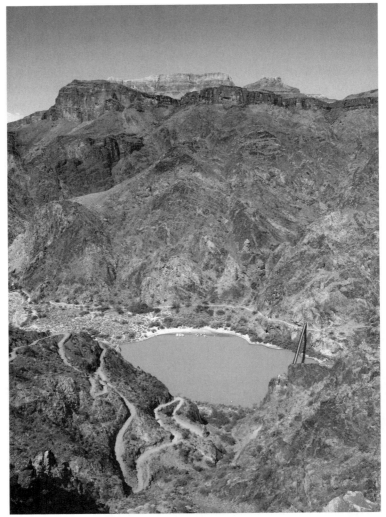

Looking down from Panorama Point, the sights include the South Kaibab Trail, Kaibab Bridge, and the mouth of Bright Angel Creek.

Soon you reach a junction. The left-hand fork is the River Trail, leading to the mouth of Pipe Creek and intersecting the trail crossing the Silver Bridge 0.5 mile downstream. The right-hand fork takes you to the entrance of a small tunnel and onto the Kaibab Bridge, also termed the black, or mule, bridge. This bridge, unlike the Silver Bridge, has a solid bottom, and the mules are willing to cross it. Head right.

**SECTION**

**7**

# Kaibab Suspension Bridge to Bright Angel Campground
Distance. . . . . . . . . . . . . . . 0.6 mile

On a hot day, this last stretch of trail is tiring. It is hot—oppressively hot—and you are simply putting one foot in front of the other trying to reach the shade of the campground or Phantom Ranch. On a cooler day you will likely spend more time enjoying the attractions. Everyone should take a brief stop to look at the Puebloan ruins by the side of the trail. I am always struck by the multitude of minute rooms that comprised Puebloan dwellings (see page 5 for more about the region's prehistoric inhabitants).

If temperatures are not too intense, you may enjoy having lunch near the trees by the side of the river. Midday during summer months you will likely share the beach with the rafts that dock on the beach to the east of the mouth of Bright Angel Creek.

A little beyond the various use trails to the beach, the trail turns to the right and you reach a junction. Straight ahead takes you to Phantom Ranch, while crossing Bright Angel Creek (on a bridge) leads to the Bright Angel Campground. Note that the sign here indicates you can continue straight ahead to the campground. There is a second bridge at the north end of the campground, but it is a longer journey.

Assuming you take the southerly bridge, you cross the creek, turn right, and walk along a path shaded by tall cottonwoods. A wall of

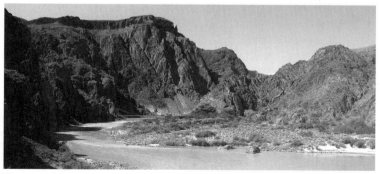

The view of the Colorado River as you cross the Kaibab Bridge

rock rises just to the left of the trail. Shortly you reach the campground: first the 2 group sites and then the 31 individual sites, with toilets at about the midpoint.

## BRIGHT ANGEL CAMPGROUND

Bright Angel Campground has 33 sites: 2 group sites at the southern end of the campground and 31 individual sites that spread from here north. Each campsite is numbered and has a picnic table, a large ammunitions box for food storage, and a pole to hang your backpack on. These sites lie along either side of the trail. With the streamside sites you have the privilege of your own piece of streamside real estate, but these sites tend to be smaller and sunnier. Most of sites on the west (nonstream) side of the trail get quite a bit of shade from the cottonwood trees. If there are still lots of sites available when you arrive, scope out the options and choose your favorite. (And don't worry, the cottonwoods lose their leaves in winter, when you want the sun.) Near the middle of the campground, there are flush toilets, as well as running water, a dishwashing basin, and even an electricity outlet. There are two water taps in the campground, one located a bit north of the toilet, and the other to the south.

This campground has more than a "natural" amount of shade, for the cottonwoods have been planted repeatedly following major floods, are surrounded by wire mesh to protect them from beavers, and are irrigated by an intricate collection of canals. Rangers and volunteers have taken much effort to ensure that this heavily used location remains lush and well maintained.

Once you establish your camp, you have many options for the remaining daylight hours. On hot days, Bright Angel Creek is full of people lying in its cool waters. National Park Service ranger programs are presented at 4 P.M. and 7:30 P.M. at Phantom Ranch—see the bulletin boards in the campground for more information. Until 4 P.M. when they close to prepare dinner, you can visit Phantom Ranch, buy yourself a cold drink, and write a postcard that will be stamped "From the bottom of the Grand Canyon." If you wish to continue hiking, see side trip suggestions on page 153.

# MAJOR LOCATIONS ON THE SOUTH KAIBAB TRAIL

| Location | GPS (UTM) Coordinates (NAD 27) |
|---|---|
| South Kaibab Trailhead | 12S 402466E 3990216N |
| Ooh Aah Point | 12S 402164E 3991115N |
| Cedar Ridge | 12S 401948E 3991427N |
| Skeleton Point | 12S 401919E 3993347N |
| The Tipoff | 12S 401906E 3994487N |
| Panorama Point | 12S 401856E 3994870N |
| South end of Kaibab Bridge | 12S 402044E 3995453N |
| Bright Angel Campground | 12S 401417E 3995553N |

| Location | Elevation (feet) | Distance (miles) | Elevation Gain (feet) |
|---|---|---|---|
| South Kaibab Trailhead | 7200 | | |
| | | 0.9 (0.9) | 600 (600) |
| Ooh Aah Point | 6600 | | |
| | | 0.6 (1.5) | 540 (1140) |
| Cedar Ridge | 6060 | | |
| | | 1.5 (3.0) | 920 (2060) |
| Skeleton Point | 5140 | | |
| | | 1.5 (4.5) | 1260 (3320) |
| The Tipoff | 3880 | | |
| | | 0.4 (4.9) | 260 (3580) |
| Panorama Point | 3620 | | |
| | | 1.3 (6.2) | 1170 (4750) |
| South end of Kaibab Bridge | 2440 | | |
| | | 0.8 (6.8) | 155 (4745) |
| Bright Angel Campground | 2490 | | |

Note: Figures in parentheses indicate cumulative information.

## Bright Angel Trail

The description for the Bright Angel Trail begins at the Colorado River, taking you up, since most people descend the South Kaibab Trail and ascend this route.

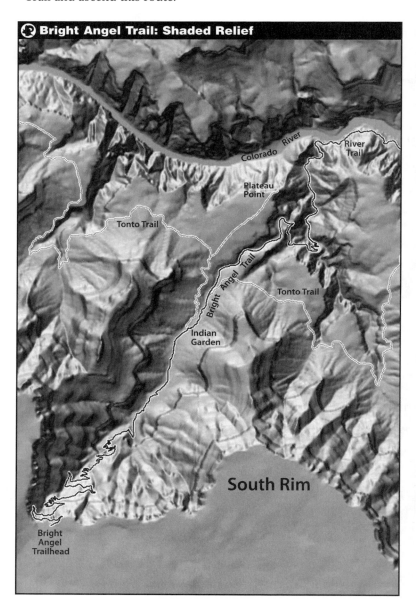

# Bright Angel Trail

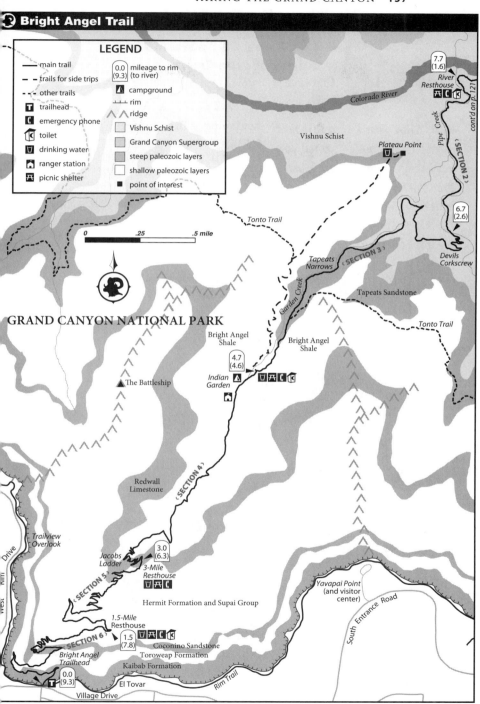

**LEGEND**

| | |
|---|---|
| ―――― | main trail |
| ‑ ‑ ‑ | trails for side trips |
| ⋯ ⋯ | other trails |
| 🚏 | trailhead |
| 🅲 | emergency phone |
| 🚻 | toilet |
| 🚰 | drinking water |
| 🏠 | ranger station |
| 🏕 | picnic shelter |

| | |
|---|---|
| 0.0 (9.3) | mileage to rim (to river) |
| ⛺ | campground |
| ⋀⋀⋀ | rim |
| ⋀ ⋀ | ridge |
| ☐ | Vishnu Schist |
| ▨ | Grand Canyon Supergroup |
| ▨ | steep paleozoic layers |
| ☐ | shallow paleozoic layers |
| ■ | point of interest |

0    .25    .5 mile

**GRAND CANYON NATIONAL PARK**

Colorado River

Vishnu Schist

Pipe Creek

7.7 (1.6) River Resthouse

cont'd on p. 121

‹ SECTION 2 ›

6.7 (2.6)

Devils Corkscrew

Plateau Point

Tonto Trail

Tapeats Narrows  ‹ SECTION 3 ›

Garden Creek

Tapeats Sandstone

Tonto Trail

The Battleship

Bright Angel Shale

Bright Angel Shale

4.7 (4.6) Indian Garden

Redwall Limestone

‹ SECTION 4 ›

Trailview Overlook

Jacobs Ladder

‹ SECTION 5 ›

3.0 (6.3) 3-Mile Resthouse

Hermit Formation and Supai Group

Yavapai Point (and visitor center)

South Entrance Road

West Rim Drive

1.5-Mile Resthouse

1.5 (7.8)

Coconino Sandstone

Toroweap Formation

‹ SECTION 6 ›

Bright Angel Trailhead

Kaibab Formation

0.0 (9.3)

El Tovar

Rim Trail

Village Drive

**SECTION 1**

# Bright Angel Campground to Mouth of Pipe Creek

Distance . . . . . . . . . . . . . . 1.6 miles

*HINT: Many Grand Canyon books refer to "river miles." When you next see such a reference, note that the Bright Angel boat beach is at River Mile 87.5 and the Pipe Creek Rapids are at River Mile 88.9 (near the mouth of Pipe Creek).*

Beginning at Bright Angel Campground, retrace your route south to the bridge across Bright Angel Creek. Instead of crossing the creek and heading east to the Kaibab (or Black) Bridge, continue west toward the Silver (or Bright Angel) Bridge. The route takes you past a large collection of park service buildings, a water tap, and a corral, before reaching the bridge. Suspended below this bridge is a large water pipe that carries water from Roaring Springs, far up the North Kaibab Trail, to the South Rim. It stays at river level until Pipe Creek and then climbs steeply to Plateau Point, on to Indian Garden, and then up to the rim. The South Rim can store enough water to last only three days.

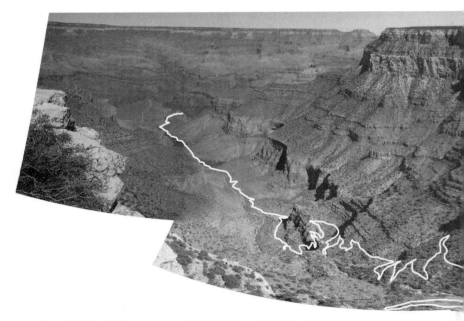

From Trailview Vista, you can see the Bright Angel Trail from the South Rim to the Tapeats

The base of the Silver Bridge is metal mesh, providing an aerial view of the swirling Colorado's waters—the mules are not fans of this and will not cross it. Halfway across the bridge is a wonderful place to look up and down the river corridor, as you are far enough from the walls to appreciate that you are in a steep gorge, above which are distant buttes. Unfortunately, except on a cool spring day, you should cross the bridge long before the sun shines deep into the gorge, limiting photo opportunities.

Across the bridge, you reach the River Trail and turn right (downstream). The left-hand direction takes you back to the base of the South Kaibab Trail and across the Kaibab Bridge. A beach of giant cobbles lies beneath the south end of the bridge, an indication of the power of the river, especially when it floods. For the first stretch you walk alongside the Colorado's banks. Shortly, you pass through a sandy expanse. Your feet slip with each step, making walking difficult. And the vegetation changes immediately, for different species are adapted to sandy substrate than the nearby rock. Water drains through the sand even faster than the rocky soils elsewhere, making it a very water-stressed environment.

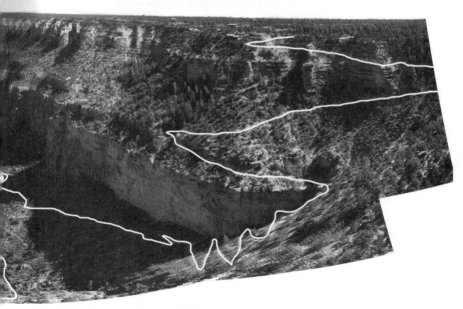

Narrows, the final 5.5 miles and 3300 feet of elevation you will cover on your ascent.

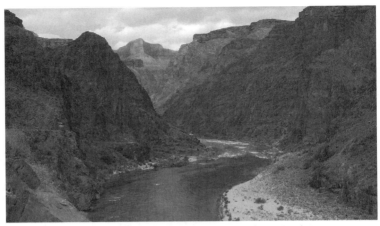

The River Trail and the Colorado River near the mouth of Pipe Creek

Beyond the sand the trail climbs slightly and you look steeply down to the river, for much of the River Trail was blasted into solid rock. You will repeatedly note that you are walking along this nearly flat four-foot-wide boulevard, but vertical walls rise above your head and fall beneath your feet to the river. The basement rocks through which you are traversing, intermingled Vishnu Schist and Zoroaster Granite, form steep, mostly dark walls on either side of the Colorado River, effectively trapping and reradiating heat on already hot days and making this stretch an oven by midmorning.

## SECTION 2

## Mouth of Pipe Creek to Where You Leave Pipe Creek
Distance . . . . . . . . . . . . . . 1 mile

*HINT: Try to escape the sun when you take a break. Even small trees and shrubs provide some shade if you sit close enough to them.*

The trail turns left 90 degrees when you reach the mouth of Pipe Creek. A resthouse and newly installed toilet are located here, but there is no water. You now begin the long climb to the South Rim. As you turn the corner and leave the banks of the Colorado, you are officially on the Bright Angel Trail. When the trail was first built, the mouth of Pipe Creek was as far as you could go, for the banks of the river were not navigable.

The first mile of uphill is one of the gentlest along the route; you climb only 330 feet as you follow the banks of Pipe Creek. The trail crosses Pipe Creek many times to avoid places where the creek abuts a cliff. And even then, much of the second half mile was blasted with dynamite. Along stretches of the creek you get to peer down to beautiful sections of polished granitic rock, while elsewhere vegetation abounds in the channel. During spring the stream is always running, but stretches of it will be dry by late summer, especially if monsoon rains are light.

## CANYON SHADOWS

When the sun is high in the sky, there is little shade in the Grand Canyon. The steep canyon walls, however, can provide shade in the morning, evening, or at times of year when the sun is at a lower angle. In the morning, west-facing alcoves and deep canyons, including the lower stretch of the Bright Angel Trail will remain shaded—even in summer. In the evening, the canyons will again be shaded. In the fall, which is still hot, and winter, north-facing sections of trail, such as the upper stretches of the Bright Angel Trail, the Devils Corkscrew along the Bright Angel Trail, Pipe Creek, and the River Trail will remain shaded except toward midday. During summer, when the heat and sun are intense, enjoy the shade of Indian Garden, along the Bright Angel Trail, until late afternoon and continue your ascent as the shadows begin to envelop the trail. Throughout the year, little shade is found on the South Kaibab Trail, a ridge route, making this a better route for descending than ascending.

To get a feel for how time of year and time of day affect the amount of shade in the canyon, explore the Google Earth "sun" feature. Google Earth, a free program you can download, shows what part of the landscape is shaded at a given time. To view the sun feature, select "sun" from the "view" menu. (Note that the terrain layer must be turned on for the shadows to display.) Then use the slider bar to change the time of day or click on the "wrench" icon to the right of the slider bar and enter a different date. I especially recommend noting the difference in shade between the summer solstice and the fall equinox, when temperatures are quite similar, but amount of shade is remarkably different.

Just before you begin the steeper climb to Garden Creek, you pass a delightful little seep that pours down the steep rock faces. Its entire path appears green compared to the surrounding desert, with the last 100-foot drop densely covered with vegetation. In spring it is adorned with flowers, especially golden columbine. If you need a quick break, detour briefly to the base.

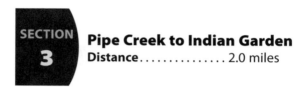

## Pipe Creek to Indian Garden
Distance . . . . . . . . . . . . . . . 2.0 miles

*HINT: The steps created by small logs are so regularly placed at two strides apart that it's easy to end up leading each stair with the same foot. If you catch yourself in that rut, stop, break your stride, and switch feet every few minutes.*

Leaving Pipe Creek behind, note the trail switchbacking persistently ahead of you. This section, known as Devils Corkscrew, takes you to Garden Creek, the drainage you will follow to the rim. The trail is well built, with a consistent and manageable grade. Small juniper logs laid across the trail prevent erosion by creating steps followed by a flat platform. With a very early start you will be able to complete much of this climb in the shade, but you will probably notice the sun encroaching downward and hope you reach the relative cool of Garden Creek, and then Indian Garden, before roasting. Throughout this stretch you are climbing through the basement rocks, where they have eroded into a steep rubble slope. The original trail descended steeply down this same slope.

Near the top of Devils Corkscrew you cross a mostly dry slickrock drainage, the same seep that feeds the little waterfall with the columbines. The trail followed this drainage, named Salt Creek, until a path was blasted through the Tapeats Narrows in 1929. Pass another small seep and shortly reach a hairpin turn. Just beyond, notice Garden Creek steeply descending a gorge. This spot is great for watching the water flow over the polished granite and imagining all the beautiful pools and cascades before the tributary merges with Pipe Creek far below.

The trail now follows the willow-thicketed banks of Garden Creek upstream. The trail crosses the creek twice in rapid succession, but mostly sticks to the eastern bank. Up ahead are steep walls— the first of the sedimentary strata, the Tapeats Sandstone. Pay close attention as you approach, noting where you cross from the truly ancient basement rocks into the only-500-million-year-old sandstone. Unlike along the South Kaibab Trail, here the Tapeats is a 300-foot-thick layer that you follow for a half mile.

*HINT: Do not head from Indian Garden (or the Tapeats Narrows) toward the rim midafternoon on a hot day. It is much wiser to take a prolonged break and begin your walk in the late afternoon, as temperatures begin to cool.*

The Tapeats Narrows, through which the trail now passes, are wonderful. The trail follows a platform, in many places blasted into the rock. The creek mostly lies below in a gorge, fairly inaccessible due to the steep rock. The rock climbs equally steeply overhead, in places overhung and occasionally forming small alcoves ideal for a break. You wind ever upward, your turns matching the river's course, until you exit onto the Bright Angel Shale. Here the creek widens and the wall of Tapeats Sandstone becomes ever shorter, until you are staring onto the quite flat Tonto Platform.

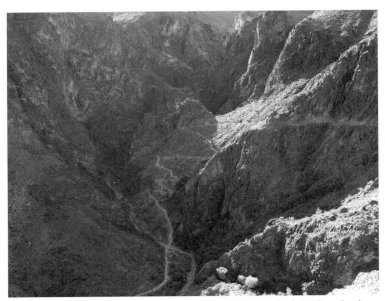

The switchbacks that comprise Devils Corkscrew climb steeply above Pipe Creek.

On the South Kaibab Trail you get a feel for the expansive Tonto Platform, but along the Bright Angel Trail, you remain first in Garden Creek's riparian corridor and then in the wash above Indian Garden and never experience the Tonto. Instead you are enjoying cottonwood trees, a thicket of grapevines, redbud trees, and maybe a few grazing mule deer. You pass a small sign for the eastbound Tonto Trail and glance at the flattish landscape it follows.

The first signs of Indian Garden are the pump house and information signs about the transcanyon water system, the impressive

## NAMESAKES ALONG YOUR ROUTE

The namesakes along the corridor trails in the Grand Canyon include names derived from Native American words and place names, the names of early visitors, and a considerable collection of whimsical names assigned by early explorers.

**The Battleship**  Named for its resemblance to a battleship.

**Bradley Point**  G. Y. Bradley was a boatman on John Wesley Powell's first expedition.

**Brahma Temple**  Brahma is the Hindu god of creation. This feature was named by geologist Clarence Dutton, who combined excellent fieldwork with artistic descriptions and creative names of the surrounding landforms. He thereby began the tradition of naming buttes and mesas for deities. Dutton also named landforms in the Grand Canyon after the other two main Hindu gods, Vishnu and Shiva.

**Bright Angel Creek**  Named by Major John Wesley Powell, honoring lines from a bible hymn that describes clear waters walked upon by angel's feet. The name was chosen to contrast with the Colorado River, named by him for its muddy waters.

**Cheops Pyramid**  Named for a pharaoh of ancient Egypt's Old Kingdom and the builder of the Great Pyramid of Giza.

**Colorado River**  Major John Wesley Powell gave the lower stretch of the river this Spanish name for its reddish color. The name has since been applied to the entire river.

setup that delivers water from Roaring Springs to the South Rim of the Grand Canyon. Around the next corner are the mule hitching posts, benches well situated beneath tall cottonwoods, a water tap, and the long row of bathrooms. If you are planning on taking only a short break, this is a perfect location; if you wish to take a longer lunch or nap, walk a few paces beyond the bathrooms and then turn right down trails that take you to a resthouse and a quieter spot beneath another grove of cottonwoods, perfect for an afternoon siesta. Hikers camping at Indian Garden need to continue about 200 feet up the trail to the sign-posted spur trail.

**Indian Garden** This land was cultivated by the Havasupai Indians until the arrival of the first European-Americans.

**Kaibab Plateau (Kaibab Trail)** The word *kaibab,* from the Southern Paiute word *Kaivavitse* that means "mountain lying down," was the tribe's term for the Grand Canyon.

**O'Neill Butte** Named for William "Buckey" O'Neill a lawyer, frontier newspaperman, and eventually a Grand Canyon prospector. With more business skills than most of his compatriots, O'Neill was able to line up funding for the long-discussed train line from Williams to the South Rim.

**Phantom Ranch** Most likely named for Phantom Creek, a tributary of Bright Angel Creek. Phantom Creek is simply an imaginative name.

**Pipe Creek** The name derives from a smoking pipe that Ralph Cameron placed along this section of the Bright Angel Trail.

**Sumner Butte** John C. Sumner was a member of John Wesley Powell's first Grand Canyon expedition.

**Tonto Platform** Named after one of the groups of western Apache, the Tonto Apache. *Tonto* derives from the Spanish word for *stupid*, and the tribe prefers to be identified as the Dilzhe'e Apaches.

**Wotans Throne** Named for Wotan, the head god (and god of war) of Germanic and Norse paganism. He is also known as Odin.

**Zoroaster Temple** Named for Zoroaster, the ancient Iranian prophet.

## Indian Garden to 3-Mile Resthouse
**Distance**. . . . . . . . . . . . . . . 1.7 miles

Beyond the Indian Garden rest facilities, you pass the campground and a ranger station. The trail is lined with tall Engelmann prickly pear cacti—a beautiful garden of color in spring when some plants display yellow flowers and others are pink. Cacti are amazing for their ability to produce such large showy flowers in a desert environment. Next you crisscross up a usually dry wash that can be dangerous in times of heavy rain. Just consider how large some of the rocks in the wash are and remember that water carried them here. Many shrubs, including apache plume, with its beautiful pink whispy seed-tails, are abundant here. A few redbud grow to the west of the wash, obvious in early spring with their abundant light

### A FAMILY STORY

In November 1966 my father emigrated from Switzerland and drove across the country to begin a job in California. En route he stopped by the Grand Canyon for a dayhike to the Colorado River via the Bright Angel Trail. A seasoned mountaineer, he carried no water, being accustomed to drinking little in the more humid Swiss Alps. He still wasn't thirsty when he left the Colorado River and began his ascent. However, by the time he was halfway back to the canyon rim, he began to look thirstily at the puddles of mule pee that dot the trail. Although he resisted the urge to sample the only available liquid, they became ever more appealing the higher he climbed.

I've heard this story since I was a child, and, knowing my father, was never sure how much the facts had been exaggerated. However, when he recently showed me his journal and it included a photo of a pee puddle, I immediately knew he had found his waterless hike out of the Grand Canyon very taxing—otherwise he would never have wasted a precious slide on unglamorous mule pee. The moral? If you aren't an experienced desert hiker, believe the experts.

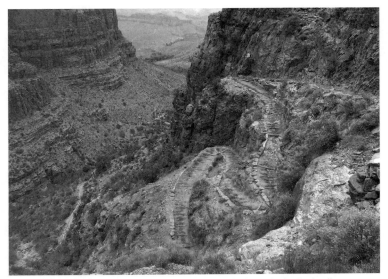

The switchbacks that comprise Jacobs Ladder climb through the Redwall Limestone along the Bright Angel Fault.

pink flowers. This entire stretch of trail is still on the Bright Angel Shale, but it erodes easily and because you are in a wash, you don't see any outcrops of it. Without a geologic map in hand, you are unlikely to notice the point you leave the Bright Angel Shale and enter the Muav Limestone, just beyond where the trail turns tightly and you begin your climb out of the wash.

**HINT: Respect the landscape. One ranger I spoke to commented that he kept coming across cacti with holes—damaged as people poked them with trekking poles. Keep your pole tips in the sand.**

The Bright Angel Trail traverses the Muav Limestone in a single long switchback and crosses into the Redwall Limestone. The latter are the rocks at which you are likely staring, for they form the steep amphitheater surrounding you. The limestone is etched and eroded by eons of water draining over it, forming alcoves and small caverns. You have undoubtedly noticed that that Redwall Limestone creates a formidable barrier most places, but here the Bright Angel Fault has offset and chopped up the rock, and the Bright Angel Trail climbs through the formation at a tight set of switchbacks referred to as Jacobs Ladder. Toward the bottom of these is a good place to observe *fault breccia*, the chopped up and cemented together jumble of rocks that form in a fault zone. The former Indian trail descended the Redwall at the same location, but dynamite was used to create such a wide trail.

At the top of Jacobs Ladder you reach the 3-Mile Resthouse. You have just climbed 1000 feet, and this is a good place for a 10-minute break with water and shade. A spur trail takes you to the resthouse and a nice vista point from which to observe the Garden Creek drainage.

## SECTION 5   3-Mile Resthouse to 1.5-Mile Resthouse
Distance. . . . . . . . . . . . . . . 1.5 miles

The landscape between the 3-Mile and 1.5-Mile resthouses is gentler, as you climb first through the Supai Formation and then enter the Hermit Formation. The landscape is more vegetated, and the ground cover of perennial and annual wildflowers can be very colorful in spring. The soil is quite red, reflecting the desert origin of the sands that comprise much of the Supai Formation. Steeper bands within the Supai indicate thicker accumulations of pure sand, and sloping sections, where silt and mud dominate. The alternating bands reflect the once changing sea level.

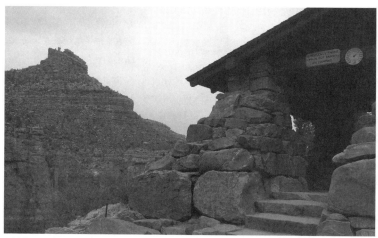

3-Mile Resthouse

As this formation is nearly 1000 feet thick, this stretch of trail can feel particularly monotonous. Stop from time to time and look down canyon for a minute, staring at the colored bands of rock surrounding you, enjoying the expanding view across the canyon, and tracing the path you've taken above Indian Garden. Just before you reach the 1.5-Mile Resthouse you enter the Hermit Formation.

SECTION 6

## 1.5-Mile Resthouse to Canyon Rim
Distance. . . . . . . . . . . . . . . 1.5 miles

Leaving the resthouse behind you have only 1.5 miles to go. This last stretch of trail is engaging, as you climb past the steep-walled Coconino Sandstone, have a chance to see Indian pictographs just below the rim, and pass through two tunnels as you complete your journey. However, there are also ever more people to contend with, as you encounter the flocks of visitors descending only slightly below the rim.

A long length of west-trending trail takes you through the Hermit Formation to the base of the Coconino Sandstone, and then up a set of tight switchbacks just east of the Bright Angel Fault. Along this stretch, the path of the fault is easy to follow because loose material has eroded from above and fills the gully. Just as the switchbacks begin, a spur trail leads to the base of the Coconino—if you have a few spare minutes, the view straight up from here is spectacular.

*HINT: The lukewarm water you're carrying may seem unappealing, but instead of replacing it with cold water at each resthouse, consider that drinking warmer water causes your body to sweat more and therefore cool itself more efficiently.*

The top of the switchbacks is the best location to note the offset between the two sides of the fault. When you reach the top of the Coconino Sandstone on the east (just beyond the "second" tunnel, since the tunnels are counted from the top), the 350-foot wall still looms above you on the west side of the fault because the Bright Angel Fault has offset the strata by nearly 200 feet. The enormous cross-bedding is readily visible in the wall of Coconino Sandstone, a reminder that giant sand dunes once covered the landscape.

Beyond the switchbacks, the trail follows the much gentler Toroweap Formation with the enormous Coconino cliff just underfoot. A long switchback through the Toroweap leads you to an often damp, lush little gully with Douglas firs. Traversing up through the Toroweap, the trail heads west, crossing the fault scarp again, thereby continuing on the passable Toroweap and avoiding the steep cliffs of the Kaibab Formation that form the wall below the rim. Turning eastward again, cross the fault and enter the Kaibab Formation. Because of the fault activity and interbedded silt layers, the Kaibab is sufficiently broken at this location to be passable.

Before you pass through the upper tunnel, stop and look at the wall above you, Mallory's Grotto. Approximately 15 feet above the trail, a beautiful panel of pictographs includes depictions of bighorn sheep. Maybe you will be fortunate enough to see actual sheep in this area; they are frequently observed along the upper stretches of

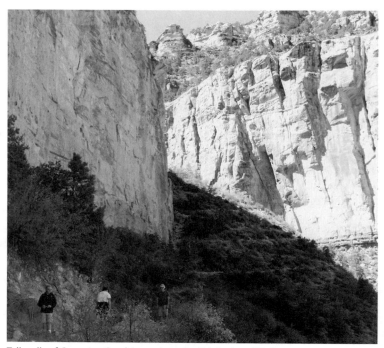

Tall walls of Coconino Sandstone along the Bright Angel Trail

the Bright Angel Trail, indeed even grazing on the grass at the top. With just a few more steps and one short switchback, you reach the top. The shuttle bus stop is just 100 feet farther, and your car is only two stops away at the Backcountry Office. Congratulations!

**Round-Trip Elevation Change**

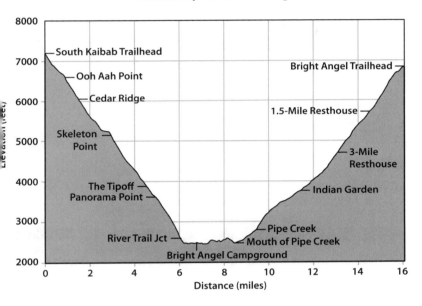

When you look at the trail's elevation profile, you will probably be surprised by how constant the gradient is, given how the landscape seems to alternate between cliffs and gentler slopes. This discontinuity between the figure and the landscape indicates the talent of the trail builders: They designed a very evenly graded trail in a heterogenous landscape. Note too how the trails across the Tonto Platform and along Garden Creek, which seem quite gentle when you traverse them, are nearly as steep as sections of "steep" switchbacks; the slope of the surrounding landscape tricks your eyes.

## MAJOR LOCATIONS ON THE BRIGHT ANGEL TRAIL

| Location | GPS (UTM) Coordinates (NAD 27) |
|---|---|
| Bright Angel Campground | 12S 401417E 3995553N |
| South end of Silver Bridge | 12S 401425E 3995063N |
| Colorado River at mouth of Pipe Creek | 12S 400019E 3995236N |
| Pipe Creek (base of the Corkscrew) | 12S 399970E 3994095N |
| Indian Garden | 12S 398568E 3993033N |
| 3-Mile Resthouse | 12S 397731E 3991602N |
| 1.5-Mile Resthouse | 12S 397464E 3991064N |
| Bright Angel Trailhead | 12S 396994E 3990678N |

| Location | Elevation (feet) | Distance (miles) | Elevation Gain (feet) |
|---|---|---|---|
| Bright Angel Campground | 2490 | | |
| | | 0.4 (0.4) | 45 (45) |
| South end of Silver Bridge | 2460 | | |
| | | 1.2 (1.6) | 190 (235) |
| Colorado River at mouth of Pipe Creek | 2480 | | |
| | | 1.0 (2.6) | 320 (555) |
| Pipe Creek (base of the Corkscrew) | 2800 | | |
| | | 2.0 (4.6) | 965 (1520) |
| Indian Garden | 3765 | | |
| | | 1.7 (6.3) | 935 (2455) |
| 3-Mile Resthouse | 4700 | | |
| | | 1.5 (7.8) | 1005 (3460) |
| 1.5-Mile Resthouse | 5700 | | |
| | | 1.5 (9.3) | 1140 (4600) |
| Bright Angel Trailhead | 6845 | | |

Note: Figures in parentheses indicate cumulative information.

# Side Trips from Bright Angel and Indian Garden Campgrounds

If you can build some spare time into your itinerary, there are several side trips worth taking from the two campgrounds. If weather and energy levels permit, Phantom Overlook, the Box, or Plateau Point make great late afternoon jaunts from their respective bases. Ribbon Falls is an all-day excursion from the Bright Angel Campground. Do not be tempted to take morning detours from Bright Angel Campground *before* beginning an ascent to the rim.

## SIDE TRIP    Phantom Overlook

see map on p. 121

**Distance:** 2.6 miles round-trip

**Elevation:** ±600 feet

**Overview:** This fairly short side trip from Bright Angel Campground is ideal either for a just-before-sunset view on the day of your descent or as a walk on a layover day. It provides a panoramic view both of the lower stretches of the South Kaibab Trail and of Phantom Ranch.

From the Bright Angel Campground, head along the North Kaibab Trail to Phantom Ranch (0.4 mile). Continue north for 0.3 mile to a signed junction. Now take the Clear Creek Trail, the right-hand fork, and begin your climb. Although less engineered than the corridor trails, this trail is less eroded because it receives much less use—it is pleasant walking. Begin by crossing a small wash filled with some gigantic boulders and then embark on an ascending traverse to a small saddle. At this saddle you will see the trail sidling across the hillside to a second, higher saddle, Phantom Overlook.

Continue on up to the overlook, and begin to take in the views as you catch your breath on the handy stone bench. The view down to Phantom Ranch is best from the point just before the bench. To avoid erosion—and injury—stay on the trail and heavily traveled areas, rather than scrambling down to the unstable rocks to remove

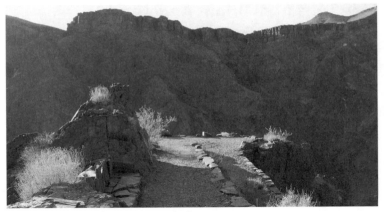

Late afternoon light at Phantom Overlook

every shrub from your view. Just beyond the bench a subtle use trail heads right, skirting a small pinnacle. Follow it for about 50 feet and you'll be rewarded with a view of the South Kaibab Trail from Panorama Point down to the Colorado River. The switchbacks are lit by the morning, but not afternoon sun.

If you wish, you can continue up this trail an additional 0.5 mile (and 500 feet of elevation) to reach the Tonto Platform.

## SIDE TRIP  Ribbon Falls

**Distance:** 12.5 miles round-trip

**Elevation:** ±1500 feet

**Overview:** This walk ends at a spectacular waterfall pouring over a tall travertine dome.

The long dayhike to Ribbon Falls is well worth the effort. You will be rewarded with a relaxing midday rest sitting on shaded platforms while admiring water spilling over a rock lip and down onto a moss-covered travertine dome. Moreover, you get to enjoy the long walk through the Box, where Bright Angel Creek runs beneath

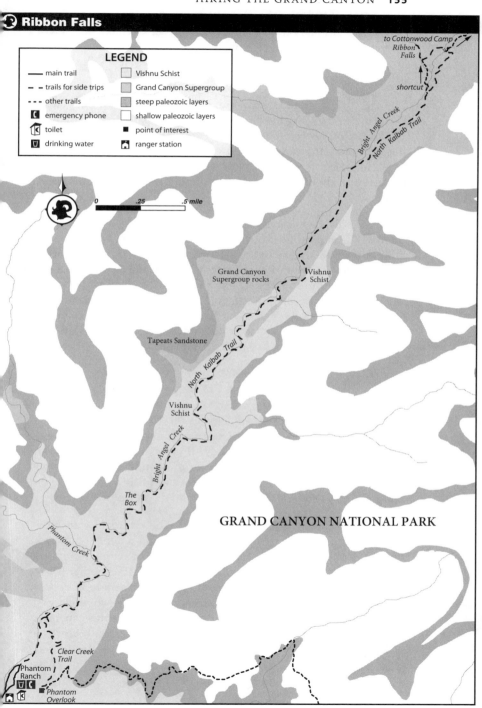

tall, steep walls of Vishnu Schist and Zoroaster Granite. Since these steep walls provide shade for many hours in the morning and evening, you can time your hike so that only the last few miles before Ribbon Falls are in the sun.

From the Bright Angel Campground head north to Phantom Ranch. Continue north along the North Kaibab Trail, pass the Clear Creek Trail junction (after 0.7 mile), and shortly reach the beginning of the Box. Here the canyon narrows and the walls become vertical. The trail skirts the east canyon wall, crosses two closely spaced bridges, and after 0.7 mile passes the junction with Phantom Creek, a slot canyon that can be explored.

There is little vegetation along the creek because, during floods, the creek occupies most of the canyon's width. The trail has been built into an amazingly flat passageway, for the water pipes carrying water for Phantom Ranch, Bright Angel Campground, and the *entire* South Rim, run beneath the trail. You are forever crossing little valves on the soil surface; note the pipe running beneath the bridges. All this work makes for fast walking and many beautiful rock walls built to protect the water system from the river. You will also notice the occasional old telephone pole.

You reach the fourth bridge after an additional 2 miles and soon afterward begin to notice that the canyon walls are starting to "descend." You are slowly climbing up through the schist and granite, approaching the overlying contact with the Grand Canyon Supergroup strata. Eventually you can see tall red walls far above—the most obvious strata is the Redwall Limestone, still more than a thousand feet above you. Continue the gentle climb and after 0.8 mile (since the fourth bridge), cross into the Grand Canyon Supergroup, as you follow a curve beyond the last of the narrows.

The change in setting is instantaneous: The riverbanks are now vegetated and the trail follows river terraces and sediment fans as it continues up a much wider canyon. Behind you the trail disappears in the narrow gorge. Meanwhile, you now see all the familiar layers of sedimentary rock rising above you; certain vantage points provide glimpses all the way to the uppermost strata, the white-colored Coconino Sandstone and Kaibab Formation. Because this canyon is broader, the sun will likely have reached you. Although hotter, the walking continues to be gentle and pleasant. The shallow desert slopes are dotted with yuccas, cacti, and shrubs. Shortly, you cross a small side creek on a bridge surrounded by reeds.

After another 30 to 45 minutes of walking you will notice that the trail climbs steeply up ahead—and that opposite (left of) this slope a side canyon merges with Bright Angel Creek. Ribbon Falls is in this side canyon and just beyond the steep slope the trail descends to a junction (1.7 miles after leaving the narrow gorge). The North Kaibab Trail continues straight ahead, while a left-hand fork takes you down to the riverbank, across a bridge, and along a use trail to the amphitheater holding Ribbon Falls. If you are comfortable with cross-country travel, a second, much shorter option requires you wade the creek. At UTM coordinates 12S 405224E 4001474N (NAD 27; or 36°9′19′′N, 112°3′13′′W), is a side trail, marked only by a suspicious line of rocks. It is about 0.4 mile before the aforementioned junction heads to the creek. This track descends to the creek, crosses where the river bottom is smooth and the willows sparse, and continues toward the mouth of the canyon. This option is not practical under high water conditions and not advised if you do not locate the start of the use trail. Many people will choose to detour north to the bridge on their way to the falls, but return on the use trail.

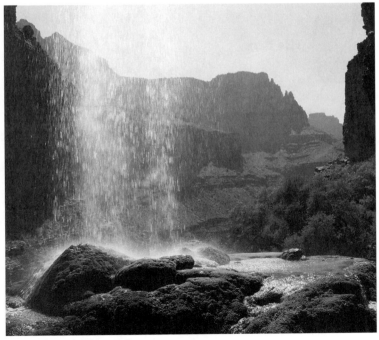

Peering through Ribbon Falls

A quarter mile from the bridge you enter the narrow, lush, shadier section of the creek. Here the trail from the bridge merges with the *alternative* route previously described. The now indistinct use trail crosses to the left (south) bank of the creek and works its way through willow thickets, up short rocky sections along the stream bank, and shortly to the base of Ribbon Falls. The water pours over a tall travertine cone. Travertine is calcium carbonate, just like limestone, and forms here because of the abundance of dissolved limestone in the water.

Walk up to the top of the falls to look down. Stand right at the base of the falls to enjoy the strangely vertical lines of moss covering the travertine cone, and poke your head inside the base of the travertine cone. Most importantly, just sit and enjoy the location. Respect the signs asking you to keep off damaged and revegetating areas. By taking a nap on one of the shaded rock platforms and sitting around until late afternoon, you can plan your descent for after the sun has left the Box.

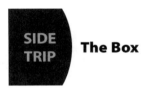

SIDE TRIP     **The Box**

see map on p. 155

**Distance:** 2.8 miles round-trip

**Elevation:** ±250 feet

**Overview:** Admire the tall walls of dark Vishnu Schist along this narrow, winding stretch of Bright Angel Creek.

If the walk to Ribbon Falls is more than you wish to embark on on your layover day, consider a journey to the Box, the narrow stretch of the North Kaibab Trail that begins 0.8 mile north of the Bright Angel Campground. Continue as far or as short a distance as you wish. Going a bit beyond the junction with Phantom Creek lets you admire the first two bridges, the elegantly built trail, and the surrounding landscape. See the Ribbon Falls description (page 154) for more information.

**SIDE TRIP**

## Plateau Point

see map on p. 137

**Distance:** 3 miles round-trip

**Elevation:** ±300 feet

**Overview:** This gentle walk from Indian Garden heads to a magnificent lookout, with views straight down to the Colorado River.

Take this walk if you are spending a layover day at Indian Garden or arrive to camp at Indian Garden with enough energy to take a 3-mile "sunset stroll." One advantage of a late afternoon walk is that you will share the trail only with other backpackers, not with the many hikers embarking on the longest of the national park sanctioned dayhikes. Avoid this side trip if thunderstorms threaten, as the entire route is exposed.

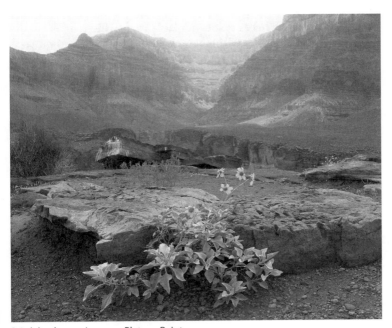

Brittlebush growing near Plateau Point

From Indian Garden Campground, retrace your route slightly downhill to the rest area and mule hitching posts. A sign here directs you west along the Tonto Trail and to Plateau Point. Paralleling the Bright Angel Trail, but on the opposite side of Garden Creek, the Tonto Trail traverses in and out of several narrow washes, before reaching a junction after 0.75 mile. Here the Tonto Trail, the much fainter of the two choices, turns west (left), while the well-traveled trail to Plateau Point continues straight ahead. For the next 0.75 mile to Plateau Point you cross a nearly flat landscape, the Tonto Platform. This walk gives you a wonderful feel of the Tonto, which exists because the Bright Angel Shale, which comprises it, is so easily eroded. The vegetation is dominated by blackbrush, named for its blackish thicket of branches that are readily visible by midsummer when its sheds its leaves. Also present are many cacti and tall century plants.

Traipse through this scenery and eventually reach a hitching post. Just beyond the trail descends slightly and ends. You turn right and scramble onto a large rock platform, the top of the Tapeats Sandstone. From here enjoy the wonderful views down to the Colorado River, observe fragments of the Bright Angel Trail, and remind yourself of your ascent, along Pipe Creek and much of Devils Corkscrew. There are lots of places from which to take in the vista, including a stretch with a guardrail—pick one based on your comfort level with exposure. Enjoy sunset from here before heading back to Indian Garden for a late dinner.

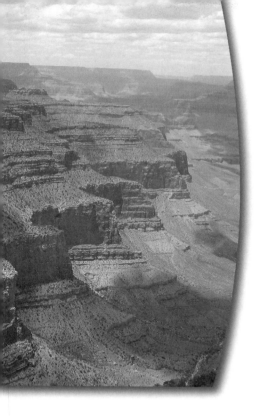

# 5

## After the Hike

**A**fter completing an ascent from the Colorado River, you are unlikely to want to embark on another hike. However, if you have some spare time, there are many (nearly) armchair activities or short jaunts to enrich your visit.

My first recommendation is to visit (or revisit) at least one of the vista points on the South Rim from which you can see your journey: Trailview Overlook for the Bright Angel Trail and Yavapai Point for both the Bright Angel and South Kaibab trails. Even if you looked down before your hike, you should revisit them now. Few people will fully perceive the lay of the land and how it relates to the trail's trajectory on their first descent into the Grand Canyon. Retrace your path, noting how the trail works its way between the rock layers. Pay attention to the boundaries between the rock layers (something that is much easier done from afar), and remember how each layer's different environments influenced your trip. Spending this extra time absorbing the landscape will enrich and solidify your

*Above:* Below Mather Point, the dissolution of Redwall Limestone has created multiple amphitheaters.

memories. In addition to its view of the trails, the Yavapai Visitor Center has great geologic displays.

If this is your first visit to the region, schedule a few extra days to visit more of the prehistoric Puebloan ruins in northern Arizona. Perhaps begin by visiting the small Tusayan Ruin (and museum) to the east of Grand Canyon Village along Desert View Drive. Walnut Canyon National Monument (6 miles east of Flagstaff on Interstate 40) and Wupatki National Monument (30 miles north of Flagstaff on Highway 89) have very impressive dwellings; visiting them takes you back in time.

A trip along the Bright Angel Trail and South Kaibab Trail will have whet the "Grand Canyon" appetite of many hikers—you may already be daydreaming about future adventures. If you have a few extra hours, you might take a shuttle bus ride toward Hermit Vista. From Hermit Vista you can view the Esplanade, a flattish shelf reminiscent of the Tonto Platform that is a sandstone layer at the top of the Supai group. And a suggestion for long after your hike: The trails you have just completed all emphasize the depth of the Grand

## GRAND CANYON LITERATURE

One of the benefits of the Grand Canyon's fame as a phenomenal location is the literature available. Whether you read it before, during, or after your own adventure, reading a well-written tale of canyon exploration allows you to visualize more of the canyon than you will see on your hike. Three worthwhile reads are John Wesley Powell's *The Exploration of the Colorado River and Its Canyons,* Colin Fletcher's *The Man Who Walked Through Time,* and Marguerite Henry's *Brighty of the Grand Canyon.* Although presented as the tale of his 1869 descent, Powell's is an amalgamation of his two descents down the Colorado River. Fletcher describes his solo adventure as the first person to walk the length of the Grand Canyon below its rim. Brighty, a children's story, is mostly based on historical characters, including Brighty the mule, who spent winters at the mouth of Bright Angel Creek and ascended to the Kaibab Plateau on the North Rim for summers. These stories represent different eras and modes of transport, but all take you deep into the Grand Canyon's mesmerizing landscape.

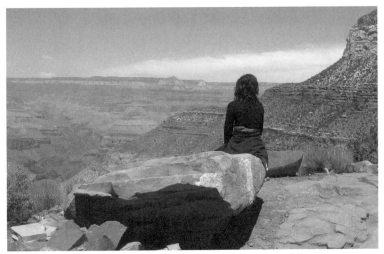

Resting on the Bright Angel Trail

Canyon, not its length and many side canyons. Return some day and hike a stretch of the Tonto Trail, maybe from the Grandview Trail to the Bright Angel Trail, to enjoy a different perspective.

The aforementioned activities keep you in tune with your surroundings, but technological attractions exist as well. Grand Canyon Airlines (www.grandcanyonairlines.com), Air Grand Canyon (www.airgrandcanyon.com), and Scenic Airlines (www.scenic.com), operating out of the Grand Canyon airport in Tusayan, provide a variety of aerial tours of the Grand Canyon. Their flights routes are east and west of the corridor trails, so you will not see your route, but of course you also didn't have to listen to their engines during your hike. Second, the IMAX theater at the National Geographic visitor center in Tusayan has a 34-minute virtual trip down the Colorado River and above the Grand Canyon. See www.explorethecanyon.com/index.cfm for more details and to buy discounted tickets in advance.

# Bibliography and Recommended Reading

## Books

Abbott, Lon, and Terri Cook. *Hiking the Grand Canyon's Geology*. Seattle: Mountaineers Books, 2004.

Anderson, Michael F. *Along the Rim: A Guide to Grand Canyon's South Rim from Hermits Rest to Desert View*. Grand Canyon: Grand Canyon Association, 2001.

———. *Living at the Edge: Explorers, Exploiters, and Settlers of the Grand Canyon Region*. Grand Canyon: Grand Canyon Association, 1998.

Berger, Todd R. *It Happened at Grand Canyon*. Guilford, Conn.: Twodot, 2007.

Blakey, Ron, and Wayne Ranney. *Ancient Landscapes of the Colorado Plateau*. Grand Canyon: Grand Canyon Association, 2009.

Butchart, Harvey. *Grand Canyon Treks*. Bishop, Calif.: Spotted Dog Press, 1997.

Coder, Christopher M. *An Introduction to Grand Canyon Prehistory*. Grand Canyon: Grand Canyon Association, 2006.

Fletcher, Colin. *The Man Who Walked Through Time*. New York City: Vintage Books, 1967.

Ghiglieri, Michael P., and Thomas M. Myers. *Over the Edge: Death in the Grand Canyon*. Flagstaff, Ariz.: Puma Press, 2001.

Grahame, John D., and Thomas D. Sisk, eds. *Canyons, Cultures, and Environmental Change: An Introduction to the Land-Use History of the Colorado Plateau*. www.cpluhna.nau.edu. Created in 2002, accessed on March 31, 2009.

Henry, Marguerite. *Brighty of the Grand Canyon*. New York City: Aladdin Paperbacks, 1953.

Houk, Rose. *An Introduction to Grand Canyon Ecology*. Grand Canyon: Grand Canyon Association, 1996.

Huisinga, Kristin, Lori Makarick, and Kate Watters. *River and Desert Plants of the Grand Canyon*. Missoula, Mont.: Mountain Press Publishing Company, 2006.

McNamee, Gregory. *Grand Canyon Place Names*. Boulder, Colo: Johnson Books, 1997.

Powell, John Wesley. *The Exploration of the Colorado River and Its Canyons.* New York City: Penguin Books (first edition, 1875), 1987.

Price, L. Greer. *An Introduction to Grand Canyon Geology.* Grand Canyon: Grand Canyon Association, 1999.

Ranney, Wayne. *Carving Grand Canyon: Evidence, Theories, and Mystery.* Grand Canyon: Grand Canyon Association, 2005.

Taylor, Therean E., and Karen L. Taylor. *Checklist of Selected Plants of the Grand Canyon Area.* Grand Canyon: Grand Canyon Association, 1992.

Thayer, David. *Checklist of the Wildlife of the Grand Canyon.* Grand Canyon: Grand Canyon Association, 2003.

Thybony, Scott. *Bright Angel Trail Guide.* Grand Canyon: Grand Canyon Association, 2004.

———. *Official Guide to Hiking Grand Canyon.* Grand Canyon: Grand Canyon Association, 2005.

———. *Phantom Ranch: Grand Canyon National Park.* Grand Canyon: Grand Canyon Association, 2001.

———. *South Kaibab Trail Guide.* Grand Canyon: Grand Canyon Association, 2006.

———. *The Incredible Grand Canyon: Cliffhangers and Curiosities from America's Greatest Canyon.* Grand Canyon: Grand Canyon Association, 2007.

Whitney, Stephen R. *A Field Guide to the Grand Canyon.* Seattle: Mountaineers Books, 1996.

# Websites

**www.nps.gov/grca:** The Grand Canyon National Park website hosted by the National Park Service is fantastic. It provides all the logistical information you need about permits, campsites, and lodging. Moreover, the multimedia section hosts numerous informative podcasts and even lectures on Grand Canyon topics (with links to YouTube videos).

**www.cpluhna.nau.edu:** This wonderful website is maintained and sponsored by several organizations, including Northern Arizona University and Land Use History of North America. It includes detailed information on Colorado Plateau prehistory and regional natural history.

**http://3dparks.wr.usgs.gov/grca/index.html:** The U.S. Geological Survey website includes a number of geology-themed photo tours in the Grand Canyon, including one titled the Phantom Ranch hike that follows the

South Kaibab and Bright Angel trails. A link at the bottom of the page accesses an online geologic map of the Grand Canyon.

**www.wrh.noaa.gov/twc/monsoon/monsoon_info.php:** The Tucson office of the National Weather Service maintains this website with information on the North American Monsoon.

**www.grandcanyon.org:** The Grand Canyon Natural History Association publishes numerous topical books. If you wish to purchase any of their books before your trip, visit this website.

**www.gchba.org:** Among other resources, the Grand Canyon Hikers and Backpackers Association hosts a copy of *The Story of David Rust,* who built the first accommodation at the Phantom Ranch location. The story was written by his grandson.

# Index

Note: Page numbers in **bold** indicate maps and photos.

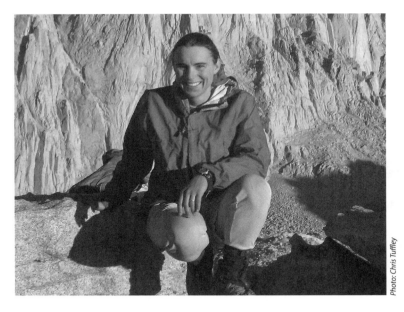

## About the Author

Since childhood, Lizzy Wenk has hiked and climbed with her family in California's Sierra Nevada and throughout the southwestern U.S. During frequent spring, fall, and winter forays into Arizona, Utah, and New Mexico she has hiked and backpacked in nearly every southwestern national park and monument. The canyon landscapes, and especially the Grand Canyon, entice her out of California again and again.

She spends her summers in the Sierra. There she has completed biology research, including her own Ph.D. thesis research on the effects of rock type on alpine plant distribution and physiology, hiked extensively for leisure, and has recently been gathering trail data for several Wilderness Press titles. Obsessed with exploring every bit of the Sierra, she has hiked thousands of on- and off-trail miles and climbed more than 500 peaks in the mountain range.

Until recently a resident of Bishop, California, she currently lives in Sydney, Australia, with her husband, Douglas, and daughters, Eleanor and Sophia. There she is beginning to explore Australia's remarkably wet and vegetated slot canyons.